Caring for Continence

A Care Assistant's Guide

Caring for Continence

A Care Assistant's Guide

Mandy Fader
Christine Norton

The publication of this book has been greatly assisted by a grant from Mölnlycke Ltd

Better Care Guides

Better Care Guides are published by Hawker Publications

First Published in 1994 by
Hawker Publications Ltd
13 Park House
140 Battersea Park Road
London SW11 4NB

Revised 1995

British Library Cataloguing in Publication Data

A catalogue record for this book is available from the British Library

ISBN 1-874790-11-6

Designed by Richard Souper

Typeset by
In Company

Illustrations and cartoons (including front cover) by Eve Morris except for Figs 6.1, 6.2, 6.3, 6.4 courtesy of Mölnlycke Ltd.

Printed and bound in Great Britain by
Cox and Wyman Ltd, Reading

Other books in this series:
Natural therapies for Older People. 1995.
ISBN 1-874790-21-3 Price: £4.50

CONTENTS

Mandy Fader RGN, BSc, Dip Ed is a Lecturer and Continence Advisor at the British Home and Hospital for Incurables and The Nightingale Institute, London. She teaches on a variety of different programmes and courses for care assistants, student nurses and qualified nurses. Her specialist subjects are continence and rehabilitation. She has worked as a research sister for the Department of Health conducting a study on incontinence pads and pants, as a community continence advisor and as senior nurse for the Continence Advisory Service in Bloomsbury Health Authority.

Christine Norton MA, RGN, BSc is Director of the Continence Foundation, and is Advisor on Continence to the Chief Nursing Officer for England. She is a former Continence Advisor in the NHS and author of a leading textbook as well as numerous articles in magazines and journals.

Preface

This book is intended for health care assistants and support workers working with adults who are elderly or disabled and live in residential settings (nursing homes, residential homes and hospital wards). We use the word *client* throughout the book to describe the people that you care for; you may call them residents or patients. For simplicity, the client is referred to as *she*, but except where indicated, the content applies to both men and women.

Although most people stay continent all their lives, incontinence is a common problem for clients in residential settings. But it is very important not to simply accept it as an inevitable part of becoming older or disabled. Our intention is to give care assistants the information they need to help clients maintain or regain continence.

Mandy Fader and Christine Norton
London 1994

1
Being incontinent

**What is incontinence? Who is incontinent?
Feelings about incontinence.
Living with incontinence.**

It is easy to take continence for granted. Most of us hardly give our bladders and bowels a second thought. We can take ourselves to the toilet when we want to and can "hang on" until we get there. But for many people, especially elderly or disabled people, continence cannot be taken so lightly. Elderly and disabled people are more likely to be incontinent than others, and this is especially true of those in residential care.

Being incontinent often results in not being able to do the things you enjoy, not being able to go out whenever you want to, worrying about smells and wet patches and what people think of you. Worst of all, being incontinent often means feeling bad about yourself.

But much can be done. Incontinence is not something that people in residential care simply have to put up with. There are ways to help clients stay continent, there are treatments to improve or even cure incontinence, and there are effective aids and equipment that can allow people who are incontinent to lead their lives with confidence and dignity.

What is incontinence?

We all know what incontinence is: it's that puddle on the floor or those soiled sheets on the bed in the corner. But incontinence is not simply passing urine or faeces (bowel motion) in the "wrong" place. The important thing about it is that the person could not help it.

Incontinence is the loss of ability to **control** the emptying of the bladder or bowel.

Being able to control the bladder means being able to do a number of **continence actions**.

To be continent you must be able to:

- **recognise** the need to pass urine or faeces
- **identify** the correct place (such as a toilet or commode) in which to pass urine or faeces
- **reach** the correct place in which to pass urine or faeces
- **hold on** until you reach that place
- **pass** urine or faeces when you get there.

If someone has a problem with any one of these actions, they are in danger of becoming incontinent.

Who is incontinent?

Anyone can be incontinent, young or old, fit or disabled. If you were travelling on a double decker bus full of people you would probably be accompanied by at least two or three other passengers who were incontinent of urine. But incontinence is more common in elderly people and in people with disabilities, and is more common in women. In fact, just the sort of people who live in residential settings. Surveys show that between a quarter and half of clients in residential homes for elderly people have urinary incontinence.

How would you feel if you were incontinent?

Think for a minute about what it must be like. Imagine you were in the supermarket and had a sudden strong urge to pass urine. You couldn't control it and there wasn't a loo in sight. You "wet yourself", wet your skirt or trousers down to your shoes. How would you feel?

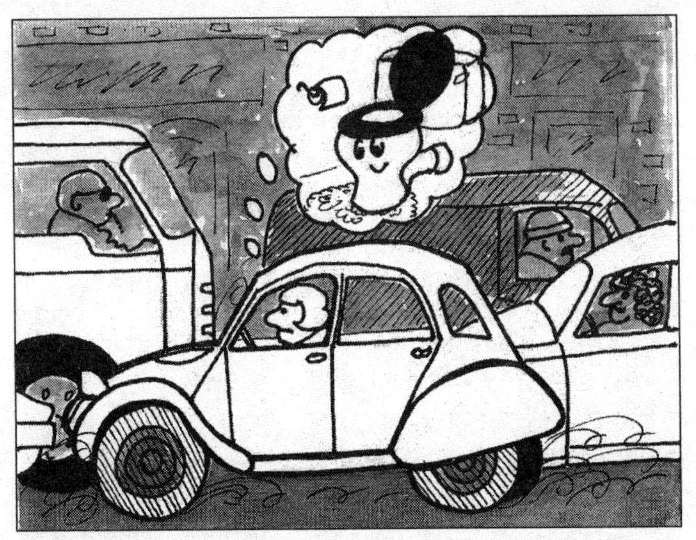

We would all be incontinent if we couldn't reach the toilet.

Perhaps, words like **embarrassed, ashamed, dirty,** or even **disgraced** came to your mind.

Now think about your clients who are incontinent. They probably have similar feelings to yours.

There can be few things more **embarrassing** than being incontinent. Being incontinent means that a very private function (passing urine or faeces) becomes very public. Many people feel **ashamed**, perhaps because we all learnt in childhood that it was "good" to be dry and "bad" to wet yourself. Shame may cause people to hide the problem, and stops them asking for help.

- About 1 in 4 women and 1 in 10 men will have an incontinence problem during their lifetime.
- Elderly people and people with disabilities are particularly at risk
- In residential homes for elderly or disabled people as many as half of clients may be incontinent.

Being incontinent day after day, night after night often leads to feelings of **helplessness** and **hopelessness.** Perhaps some of your clients seem **resigned** to being incontinent. It may even seem that it just doesn't bother them anymore. But, if people don't show their feelings, it does not meant that they are happy about being incontinent. You may "get used" to having toothache and not complain about it, but it doesn't mean you don't wish it would go away or wouldn't feel much better without it. Many people come to **accept** being incontinent because they think that nothing can be done. Eventually it is quite common for people to become **depressed**.

What about your feelings?

Of all the care that you give to clients, dealing with urine or faeces is probably near the bottom of your list in terms of being pleasant or enjoyable. A lot of carers feel **distaste** and sometimes **disgust** about clearing up incontinence. You may also feel **embarrassed** about doing such things as wiping people's bottoms or helping to clean up clients of the opposite sex. But most of us learn to put these feelings aside and "get on with the job".

In practice this means that incontinence is often managed with neither carer nor client mentioning it. This may help to spare everyone's feelings, but it means that incontinence may never be talked about frankly and openly.

It is easy to see then how incontinence becomes **accepted** as "normal" and inevitable, without thinking about what might be causing the incontinence and what could be done about it.

Perhaps you have also felt **angry** and **frustrated**. Why couldn't the client wait until you brought the commode? Why is that client wet again, when you only changed her an hour ago? Understanding **why** people are incontinent can turn these feelings into more positive action.

Some carers feel **guilty** about incontinence in the

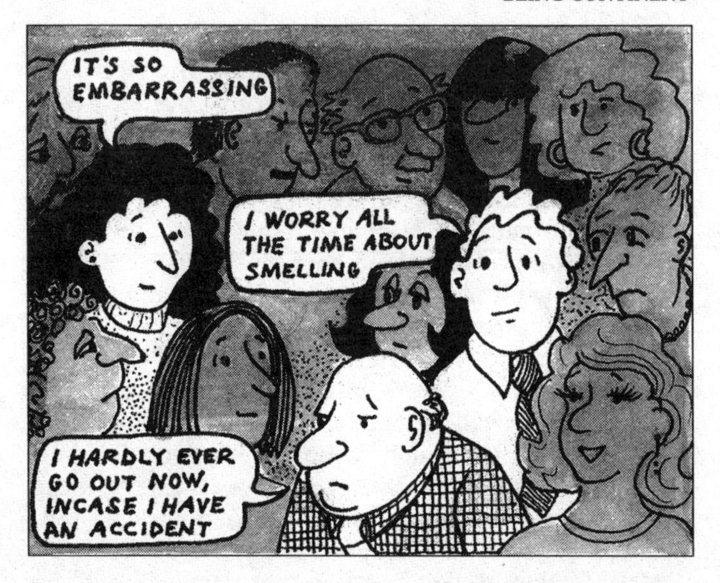

places they work in. Is it "bad nursing care"? Have they simply failed to prevent it? Could all clients be continent if only the staff tried hard enough? The answer is "No". Although much can be done (and the aim of this book is to help you to do it), not everyone can be continent despite our best efforts. The goal is to help clients be as continent as possible, given their individual problems .

Living with incontinence

Incontinence not only affects the way people feel about themselves, but it also affects the way they lead their lives. Living with incontinence often means that people make important changes in the social side of their lives.

Think for a minute about your own interests and social life; then think again about how incontinence might affect these activities. Perhaps you like to play sports, go to the pub, go on holiday, do gardening, go to bingo, visit friends and relations, have parties... the list could go on and on. But wouldn't all these things be much more difficult if you were incontinent?

Like you, clients will (or would like to) have their own interests and social life. But being incontinent is a great barrier to taking part in enjoyable activities. Staying with relatives for Christmas or visiting friends may seem impossible because of worrying about having an "accident". **Going out** just about anywhere can be stressful; fear of getting "caught short" prevents many people from going to places and joining in social events.

Journeys are often particularly worrying: "When will the coach stop?", "How will I use the toilet on the train?" "Where will I change my pad?" It's not surprising that many incontinent people simply restrict their journeys to nearby places they know well and to those where the toilet arrangements are tried and trusted. Many people of course, simply don't go out at all.

Making friends and meeting new people is difficult if you are concerned about such personal things as smells and wet patches. Fear of discovery, embarrassment and rejection may be so strong that close (and intimate) relationships are avoided.

Being incontinent is a **physical** problem that affects the way people feel about themselves (their **psychological** health) and the way they lead their lives (their **social** health) perhaps more than any other physical problem. For this reason improving incontinence and helping people to cope with living with incontinence has to be one of the most rewarding and worthwhile aspects of any care assistant's work.

KEY POINTS

- Incontinence means being unable to control passing urine or faeces.
- To be continent you need to be able to do five continence actions.
- Incontinence is a common problem, particularly for people in residential settings.
- People who are incontinent often feel ashamed and embarrassed.
- Many incontinent people think that nothing can be done, which can mean they feel helpless, hopeless and alone.
- Clearing up incontinence is an unpleasant job for care assistants.
- Incontinence often stops people from going out and joining in social activities.
- Much can be done to improve incontinence and enable people to lead a “normal” life.

2
Staying continent

Coming in to home or hospital. Communicating needs. User-friendly toilets, and alternatives. Clothes. Routines. Help with toileting. Privacy. Staying mobile. Eating and drinking. Surroundings, reality orientation.

Becoming incontinent doesn't usually happen suddenly. Problems that interfere with a client's ability to be continent often develop gradually. Preventing these problems whenever possible and providing care and surroundings that encourage continence is the basis for helping clients to stay continent.

Remember that to be continent you must be able to:
- **recognise** the need to pass urine or faeces
- **identify** the correct place (such as a toilet or commode) in which to pass urine or faeces
- **reach** the correct place in which to pass urine or faeces
- **hold on** until you reach that place
- **pass** urine or faeces when you get there.

Coming in to a home or hospital

The period of time immediately following admission is a "risky" time for continence. Moving house is a stressful event for anyone. And when that house move means giving up a home that you may have lived in for many years, for a much larger home full of strangers and unfamiliar routines and surroundings, this can be a severe blow.

Many people take a long time to adjust to moving into residential care, and it is during the first few days or weeks after admission that a previously continent person can easily start to become incontinent.

Unfamiliar surroundings can mean that a new client can have trouble knowing exactly where they are, feel muddled and may have difficulty remembering where the toilets are even though they may have been shown them several times. Sometimes this may be because the toilets may not be clearly marked.

A new client may also feel **embarrassed** about asking for the toilet, or embarrassed about sharing toilets or using the toilet facilities provided (such as a commode). He or she may simply "hang on" until it is too late.

Different routines can easily put a person out of sorts and cause **strain** and **anxiety**. Being anxious often affects the bladder and bowels and tends to make them more irritable (most of us find that we are "in and out" of the toilet at anxious times, such as before a driving test or job interview). This can mean that the client has difficulty **holding on** and **reaching** the toilet in time.

All these things, often combined with a disability or mobility problem, such as arthritic joints, can add up to a new client having **temporary** problems with staying continent. But these problems will often pass and can be greatly helped by sensitive and discreet attention to toileting needs, and by helping clients adjust to their new surroundings.

Accepting and **expecting** incontinence at this stage ("Oh, don't worry about that, lots of people here have problems with wetting, we're used to it") can mean that the client thinks that incontinence is inevitable and that nothing can be done to prevent it.

Be confident and hopeful; most clients who are conti-

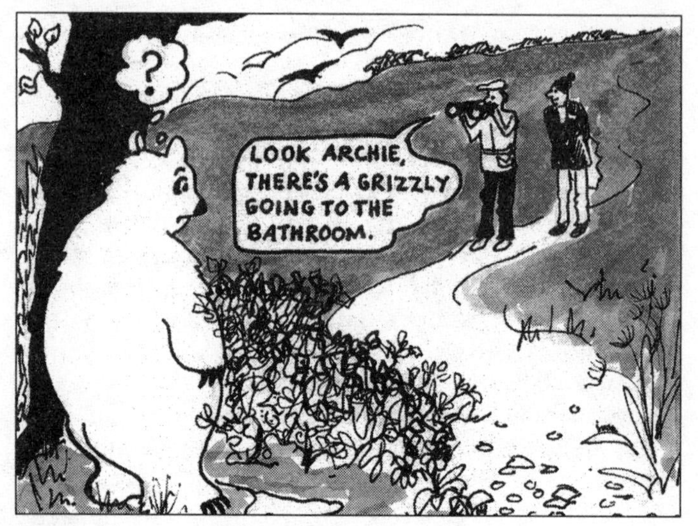

People like to use different words for the "toilet".

nent before admission can remain continent (despite a few "accidents") if attention is paid to their continence needs.

Toileting

Staying continent in residential care often depends to a great extent on the way toileting is carried out and and on the toilet facilities provided. Finding out about the client's own feelings and preferences and finding out what toileting needs she has is an important step.

Toileting preferences and needs

- **How** does the client **communicate** toileting needs?
- **Where** does the client prefer to pass urine and faeces?
- **What** additional toilet aids and/or clothing adaptations are needed?
- **When** does the client usually like/need to use toilet facilities?
- **What help** is needed from care assistants?

How does the client communicate toileting needs?

Clients who depend on you to help them get to the toilet or to bring an alternative toilet facility to them, will need to communicate these needs to you. It is important that both you and the client have a common understanding of the words that are used. Different people have different terms for words like "toilet", "urine" and "faeces". Find out what the client means and ensure that she understands what **you** mean. If possible use the words that the client is most comfortable with (see Glossary page 88).

If the client cannot communicate with words then you will need to find another way for her to let you know that the toilet is wanted. Help may be needed from a speech and language therapist, but you may be able to find out ways that the client can communicate: Can she read or write? Can she recognize a picture of a toilet? Can she blink or move her eyes in a certain way? Sometimes the client may pull at her clothes, fidget or behave in a particular manner that shows that she needs to use the toilet. Once you have identified any actions be sure to tell the senior staff so that notes can be made in the care plan or client's notes.

Clients who cannot communicate their toileting needs because they are confused may need you to be able to anticipate when they need to use the toilet. A confused client may have difficulty **recognising** that they need to pass urine or faeces or have difficulty being able to **identify** the toilet.

If clients are taken to the toilet at times when they do not really feel the need to pass urine, then they may start to forget what the toilet is for; the connection between a full bladder, the toilet and passing urine may become lost.

Finding out when a confused client is likely to want to pass urine is important to help them stay continent. This can be achieved by **charting** and forming an **individualised toileting programme** (see chapters 4 and 5).

Where does the client prefer to pass urine and faeces?

As most of us will spend most of our lives passing urine and faeces in a toilet, then a toilet is probably the preferred place to do so in residential care. But for some clients alternatives to the toilet may be easier and the client may find an alternative facility preferable.

Loos, lavatories and toilets

Are you fussy about toilets? When faced with a row of toilets do you look from one to another until you find one that you want to use? Would you rather "hold on" and wait until you get home than use a dirty toilet? Everyone is different and some of us don't give two hoots about the toilet we use. But many of us are very particular and feel anxious and unhappy about using toilets that don't meet our own standards.

Think for a minute about what is important about a toilet that makes it "user friendly" for just about everyone.

You may have included similar suggestions to these below:

Clean	**Dry seat**
Soft toilet paper	**Flushed**
Paper easy to reach	**Warm**
Hand washing facilities	**Private**
Lockable door	**Good ventilation**
No queues	**No smell**

If you had mobility problems or other disabilities, or were dependent on care assistants to take you to the toilet, you would probably need to add to the list:

Close by	**Call or help buttons**
No obstacles (such as stairs)	**Clearly signposted**
Easily opened door	**Grab rails**
Room to turn a wheelchair	**Non-slip floors**
The right height	

Take a look at the toilets provided for clients and staff in your home to see if their needs are being met. You may well find that the staff toilets seem to be satisfactory but the client toilets fall short on some points. Most of the important points of a "user-friendly" toilet listed

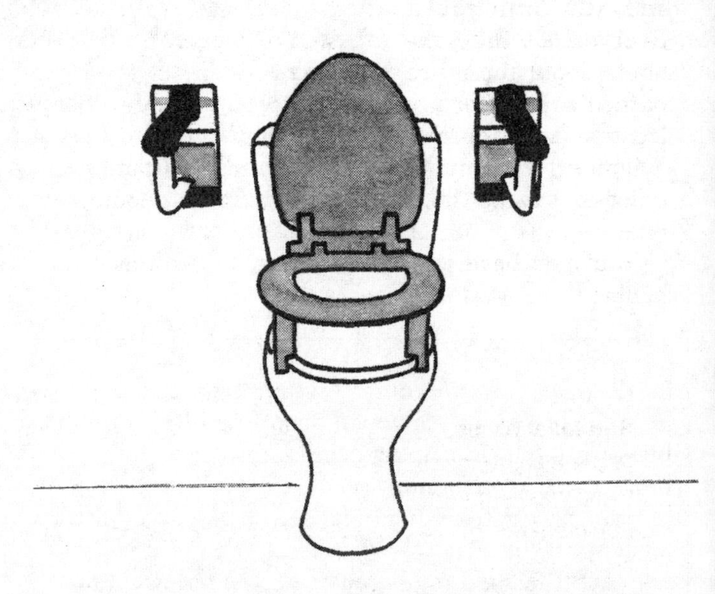

Fig 2.1 Raised toilet seat with hinged grab rail on wall.

above can be achieved without great change or expense. Providing more toilets or making them larger so that a wheelchair can be moved around in them is more difficult, but your manager should be told about such problems so that changes can be considered for the future.

What additional toilet aids and/or clothing adaptations are needed ?

Providing the right toilet aids requires careful thought. Different clients will have different needs so be sure that any aids (such as a raised toilet seat) are adaptable. Toileting won't be helped if the aids get in the way or make the client feel less secure rather than more. Balancing shakily on a raised toilet seat can put any short person off going to the toilet altogether!

Toileting aids

Grab rails – these may be fixed or hinged (so that they can be lifted out of the way) (Fig 2.1).
Raised toilet seats – enable people with stiff or painful joints to sit down on the toilet and get up with the least discomfort or effort. Some have armrests (Fig 2.1).
Padded seats – padded seats increase comfort and reduce pressure on the skin; they are particularly useful for thin people or people who need to sit for a while to be able to pass urine or faeces.

Why are "user-friendly" toilets so important?

Looking back to the things that are necessary for continence it is easy to see why a "user-friendly" toilet has a big part to play in helping people stay continent.

Because if you cannot:
identify the toilet (eg because you can't read the signpost) or
reach the toilet (eg because it is too far away) or
hold on (eg if there is a queue) or

pass urine or faeces (eg because lack of privacy is making you anxious)
you are at risk of being incontinent.

Alternatives to the toilet

Some people may prefer a commode or perhaps a bedpan or urinal to a toilet, particularly at night. Indeed for clients who have problems **holding on** or **reaching** the toilet in time these can often be a real benefit as they can be provided more easily and speedily and therefore prevent incontinence.

The main aim of alternatives to the toilet is that they in some way make toileting easier for the client, but it is also essential that they are acceptable. **Any** other toilet facility that a client is not used to can cause anxiety (have **you** tried to pass urine on a bedpan?) so their use should be discussed with the client first. Explain how it works and what the client has to do. You might find it surprising but a lot of people don't know what to do with a bedpan or a bottle!

It is also worth remembering that the same "user-friendly" things matter as much for a bedpan or commode as they do for a toilet. In particular the facility should be clean and clients should have the opportunity to wash their hands if they want to. People have different views regarding hygiene, and clients from some cultures and religions may want to wash other parts of their body or need to follow a particular hygiene ritual. Ask your clients what their wishes are.

Some toilet alternatives are made for everyday use, but others are intended for more special events such as holidays, journeys and trips. It is often best to have a practice run with any alternative that is intended for a journey or holiday. This ensures that the client can use it successfully and helps to give confidence and reduce anxiety. A travel rug is a useful addition for any journey,

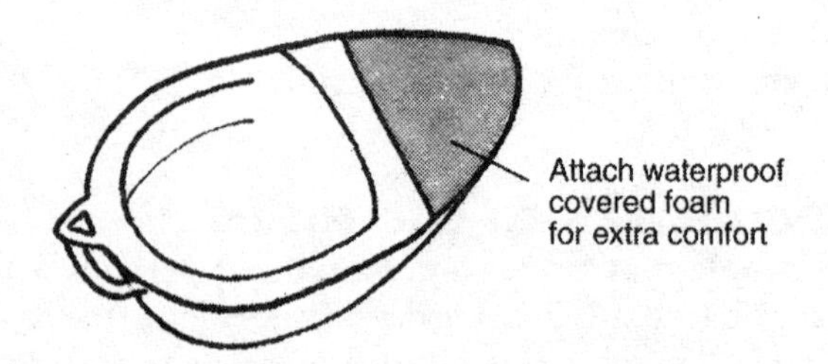

Fig 2.2 Slipper bedpan.

so that urine can be passed discreetly underneath it.

Commodes - a wide range of commodes is available and some have features such as removable armrests (for sideways transfer from bed or wheelchair), wheels and footrests. Others can be wheeled over the toilet and used as a sanitary chair.

Generally a commode is easier to use and more successful than a bedpan, and should be used whenever possible. But if the client is incontinent **as** she gets out of bed at night or is unable to get out of bed without a great deal of trouble and effort (due to disabilities) then a bedpan or female urinal is better.

Bedpans - slipper bedpans (Fig 2.2) tend to be more

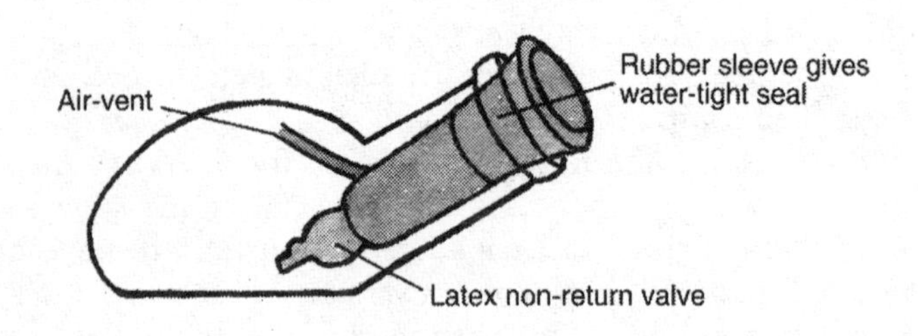

Fig 2.3 Male urinal with non-spill adaptor.

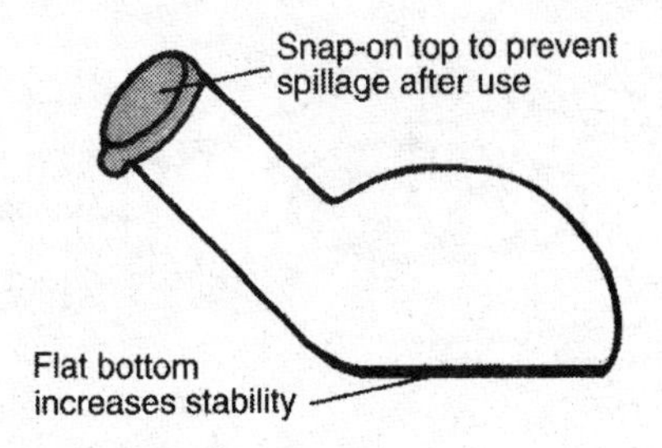

Fig 2.4 Flat-bottomed male urinal.

comfortable and easier to use than ordinary bedpans.

Male urinals (bottles) - ordinary bottles (Fig 2.3) may spill over if used in the bed overnight; flat-bottomed urinals help to overcome this problem (Fig 2.4). Disposable urinals are much more discreet than other bottles and are best for trips and journeys (Fig 2.5). An extra plastic bag that is strong and sealable (like a freezer bag) may be used to keep the used disposable bottle in until it can be discarded.

Non-spill adaptor - (Fig 2.3) fits into the neck of male urinals and stops urine from spilling out if the urinal slips out of position or is knocked over. Make sure that it fits snugly into the neck of the bottle and that the air vent is not pointing down into the urine.

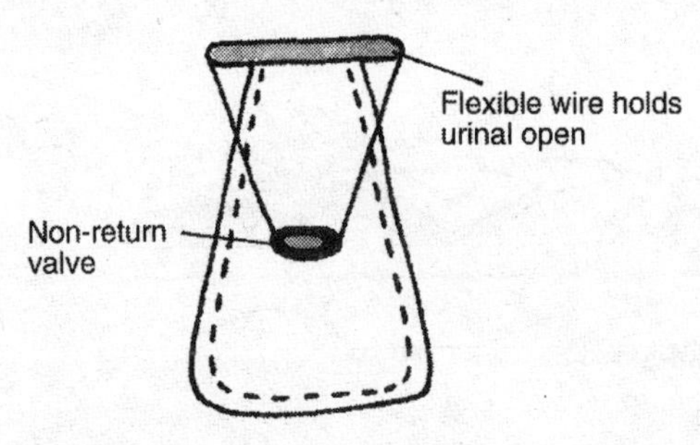

Fig 2.5 Disposable male urinal.

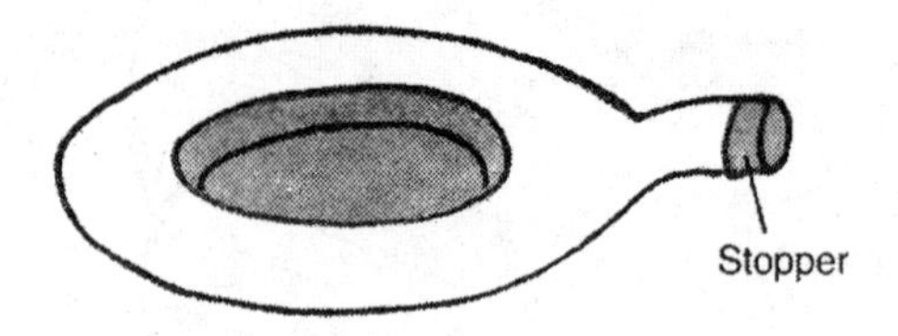

Fig 2.6 Pan type female urinal.

Female urinals - such as the "pan type" urinal (Fig 2.6) can be used by the client herself in bed (and therefore encourage independence) or can be used by care assistants as an alternative to the slipper bedpan.

The swan-necked urinal (Fig 2.7) may be even easier to use for some women. Both these are small compared to normal bedpans and may be useful for taking on holidays.

Most female urinals are difficult to use in a wheelchair. However the Bridge urinal (Fig 2.8) is designed for wheelchair use and the St. Peter's boat (Fig 2.9) may be used if the wheelchair has a cut away portion at the front and the client is able to move forward a little.

Gel powder sachets - can be put into any urinal, bed-

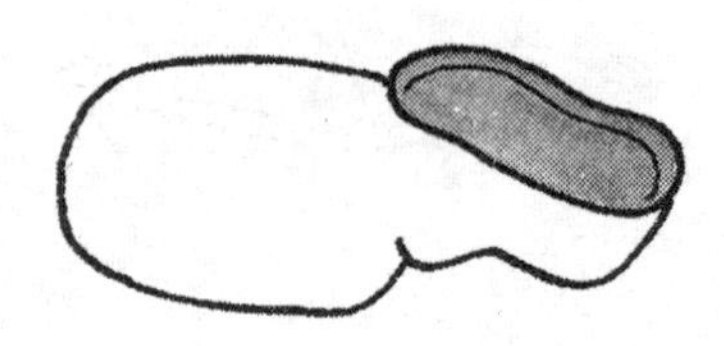

Fig 2.7 Swan-neck female urinal.

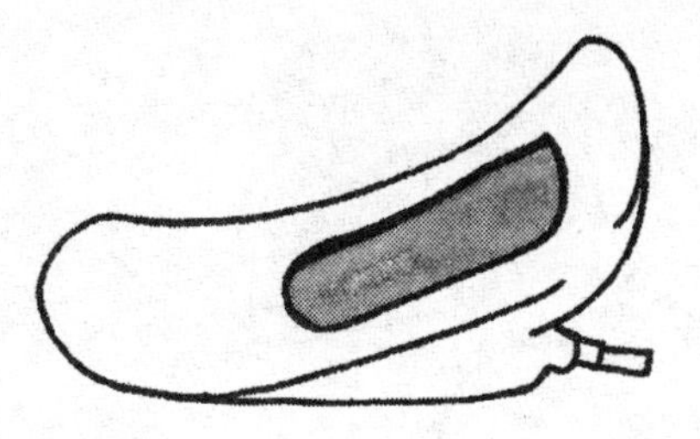

Fig 2.8 Bridge urinal.

pan or commode to prevent spillage. As the powder mixes with the urine it forms a firm jelly which will not spill and can be easily washed away.

Clothing adaptations

Providing toilet alternatives and extra aids to help with toileting is only half the battle if clothing gets in the way. It may be possible to buy special clothes for a client or adapt their own clothes in some way, but clothing choices are very personal and you will need to talk this over with the client. It is usually easier to offer different clothing or adaptations as a "trial" so that clients can get used to the change, but will feel that they can always go back to what they used to wear if they are unhappy.

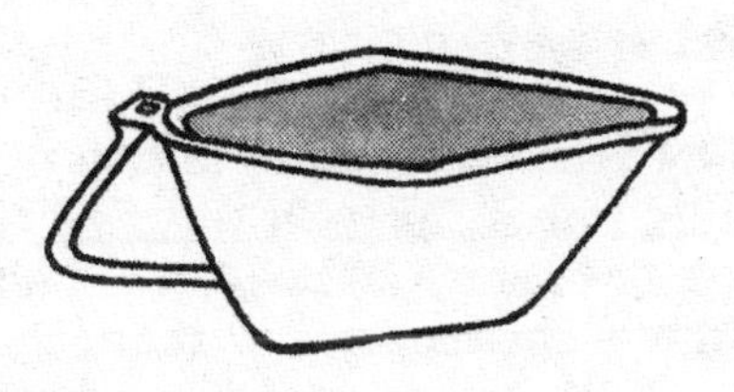

Fig 2.9 St Peter's boat.

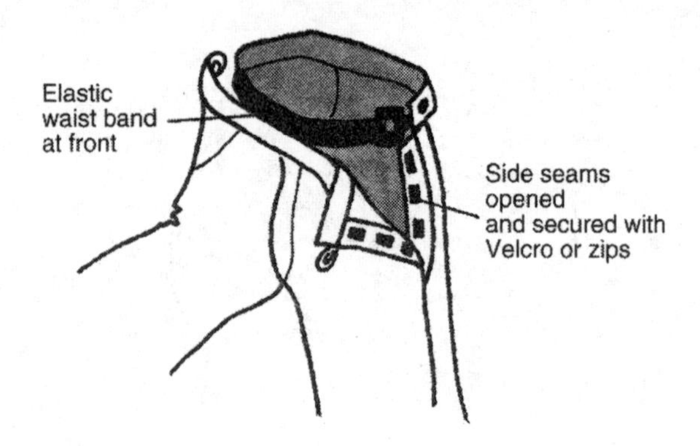

Fig 2.10 Drop front trousers

Remember that many people need a lot of practice getting used to any clothing adaptations (or toilet aid or alternative) so don't be too hasty in abandoning them. Give them a fair trial.

Replacing fly zips with longer zips can be a very useful adaptation for men using a urinal during the day. A longer zip makes it much easier to pass urine in a bottle while sitting down.

Zip pulls – enable the person to get a much better grip on a zip and are helpful on flies, particularly if the client has poor use of one or both hands.

Velcro dabs – can be used to replace zip flies, but may cause problems in the laundry (they gum up with fibres). So make sure that the velcro is closed together before sending to the wash.

Drop-front trousers – can be helpful for men or women to allow access for a urinal in a chair (Fig 2.10).

Front-opening pants - prevent the need to pull pants down and up. The pants can be undone and left on the chair when the client transfers to the toilet (including with a hoist). They can be used in conjunction with a split back dress or nightie (see below). Front opening pants may also allow for the client to pass urine into a

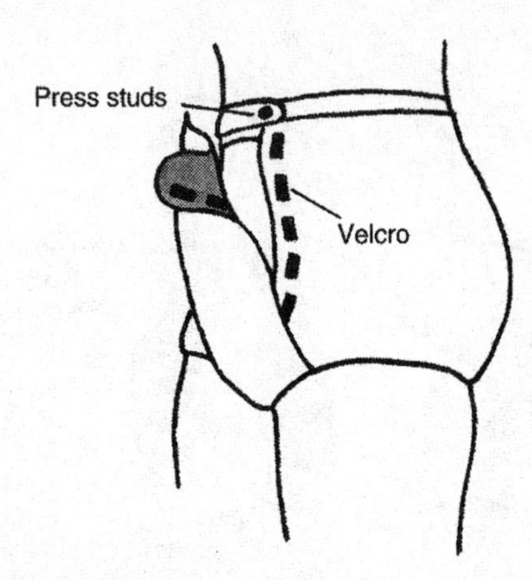

Fig 2.11 Drop-front pants

urinal while staying seated in a chair or wheelchair (Fig 2.11).

French knickers, "gussetless" pants or crotch fastening pants – all allow for urine to be passed without taking pants off. But some people don't find them acceptable at all (Fig 2.12).

Split-back dress, skirt or nightie - prevents skirts or nighties from needing to be pulled up for toileting or

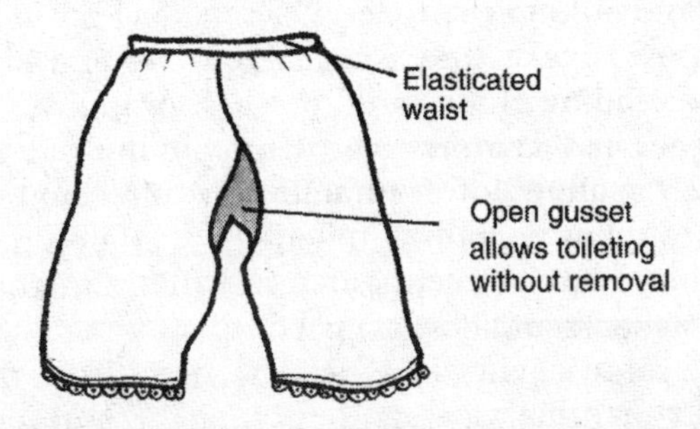

Fig 2.12 Gussetless pants.

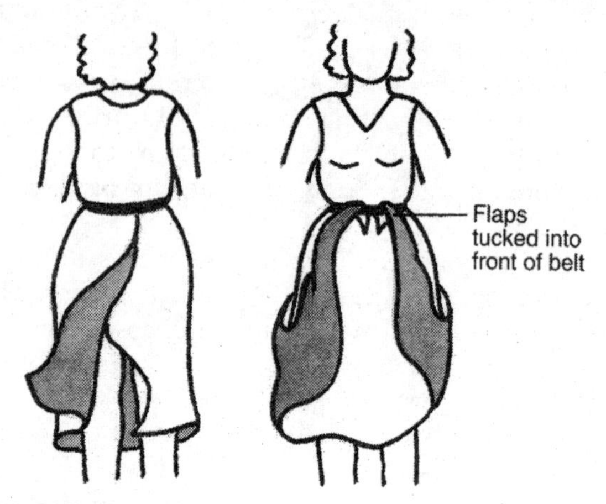

Fig 2.13 Split-back skirt.

using a bedpan. Make sure that there is plenty of overlap (at least 7 inches) at the back so that the client's bottom is always covered. For this reason these should not be used for clients who walk as there is always a risk that they can open up at the back (Fig 2.13).

When does the client usually like/need to use toilet facilities?

Routines

Most of us go to the toilet when we feel the need to go and some of us have particular routines and habits that we are used to. But it is all too easy for individual toileting needs and routines to be disrupted in residential care by the "routine" of the home. It is often more convenient to do a "round" of toileting at certain times in the day than to take clients at times that suit them (and their bladders and bowels) personally.

But some clients may need to pass urine more frequently than the toileting times on offer, and may therefore be incontinent. Others may not need to go so often and may not use the toilet when they arrive; toileting is then frustrating, wastes staff time and puts the client at risk of losing the important connection between a full bladder, sitting on the toilet and passing urine. Meeting clients' individual needs will help them to stay continent. (More on **individualised toileting programmes** in chapter 5.)

For many people the urge to pass faeces occurs after eating food, often in the morning shortly after breakfast, and it is a good idea to offer toileting assistance at this time. Constipation easily occurs if the urge to pass faeces is allowed to pass by without the opportunity to open bowels on the toilet.

What help is needed from care assistants?

Generally speaking clients should be encouraged to do as much as possible for themselves, but help may be required in one way or another from a care assistant. Very disabled clients may need help in all aspects of toileting. As with every aspect of the care that you give to clients it is important that everyone sticks to the client's own plan of care. Whatever aids are required and whatever help is needed, this should all be agreed with the client (whenever possible) and written in the care plan or client's notes (and then read!) to ensure that the care is consistent.

Privacy and embarrassment

Using the toilet is an extremely personal and private activity. Many of us find using the toilet difficult if we feel that someone might be able to hear us or notice any smell. Being watched would be even worse! But in residential care this can easily happen. It may be easier to wait with a client while they use the commode than to come back for it later. Suddenly this private activity becomes a public one, and this often causes embarrassment and anxiety. These feelings, in turn, may make it

Ensuring privacy and reducing embarrassment

- **Ask** the client about their toileting needs quietly (don't tell the world!)
- **Close** doors (making sure that the client has a call button).
- **Close** curtains carefully so that there are no gaps.
- **Busy** yourself with something (if you need to be present).
- **Run** a tap (this provides some noise and may help the client to pass urine).
- **Turn** on a radio or television.
- **Give** the client a room spray (to help with odour problems).

difficult for a client to pass urine or faeces when they are on the toilet. The client may also feel so embarrassed about being toileted that he or she may put off going until they are no longer able to hold on. Incontinence can then result.

Probably the greatest help that you can give to a client who needs help with toileting is to ensure their **privacy** and help to reduce their **embarrassment.** How can this be done? You probably have many ideas of your own. A few suggestions are listed in the box above.

Although most people want privacy while they use the toilet, some people may want or need you to stay with them. This is fine but it is still important to pay attention to ensuring privacy generally, as explained above, and to reduce embarrassment which the client may still feel.

Help may also be necessary to remove clothes and to enable the client to get comfortable on the toilet. Remember that **time** as well as privacy is important for passing faeces. If the client feels she is being hurried she may well put off passing faeces until another time, and constipation may result.

When leaving the client ensure that she knows when you will return and has some means of calling you (such as a call button). Once you get busy doing other things it is easy to forget all about the client you left on the toilet. This is not only upsetting for the client, but also dangerous. The client may try to get off the toilet and fall; pressure from the toilet seat is bad for the circulation to the skin over a long period of time and frail clients may easily become cold.

Clients may also become (understandably) angry about being left on the toilet for a long time; they may even become aggressive. After a bad experience the client may feel worried about using the toilet again (and this of course, may mean that she becomes incontinent).

Staying mobile

Being mobile and independent means that incontinence is less likely. Surveys have found that people who are mobile on their feet are not only less likely to be incontinent of urine than people who are immobile, but also have less severe incontinence if this occurs. Walking also helps to prevent constipation which can play an important part in incontinence of urine and faeces (see chapter 3). Being active and moving around stimulates the bowel to move faeces along so that constipation is less likely. You may have experienced constipation yourself as a result of not being active, perhaps if you were ill in bed or had an injury that stopped you moving about.

Walking aids such as a stick, tripod or frame can greatly improve mobility, but just as importantly, so does practice. If walking is not encouraged or expected and the client spends most of her day sitting down, then gradually walking becomes more difficult as joints become stiffer and muscles weaker. The client can also lose confidence in her own walking ability which may then make her reluctant to walk and so a vicious circle begins. Supportive shoes are vital for walking, and sloppy slippers should be avoided as these can limit walking practice and may be dangerous.

Walking to the toilet is usually a good idea, but if the client needs to use the toilet quickly then it is often better to speed her there in a wheelchair than risk incontinence. The client can always walk back from the toilet when her bladder or bowel is empty.

For clients who use wheelchairs because they are unable to walk, making the surroundings and particularly the toilets suitable for moving and turning a wheelchair is important. Some wheelchairs can "turn on a sixpence" and this is useful when space is limited.

Drinking

People who are worried about becoming incontinent (and those who are already incontinent) often cut down on the amount they drink in an attempt to prevent or reduce the problem. We need to drink at least 1-2 litres (2 - 4 pints or 8 cups) of liquid every day.

But the timing of drinks can be adjusted to suit the client. If, for example, the client needs to get up and pass urine twice or more at night then most of the fluids can be taken during the daytime and less drunk in the evening or at night. It is usually best to avoid any hard and fast rules such as "no drinks after teatime".

It can be difficult to ensure that clients do drink enough and for this reason it is important to find out what they like to drink and provide it. A pint of beer can slip down very easily for those who like it, but it is prob-

Too little liquid can:

- **lead** to dehydration and cause confusion
- **reduce** the amount of urine the bladder can hold
- **produce** strong urine which can irritate the bladder or urethra
- **make** urine infection worse
- **make** constipation worse.

ably better drunk in the daytime or early evening than last thing at night!

Some people find that tea, coffee or alcoholic drinks "go straight through them" so alternative drinks may be preferable, particularly when toileting might be a problem, such as when going on a journey.

Ensuring that clients drink enough liquids is important in preventing constipation. If liquid intake is low then faeces can easily become hard and dry (water in faeces makes it soft) and difficult to pass.

Generally people at risk of incontinence tend to restrict their drinking, but some people drink very large amounts. Sometimes this is because they were once told to drink a lot to "flush out the bladder" and have kept the habit. Drinking very large amounts (4 litres or more) can contribute to incontinence; a slow programme of fluid reduction (drinking one cup less a day for a week, then two cups and so on) may be useful. People who have drunk large amounts daily for a long time often find it difficult to suddenly change the habit.

Eating

It has long been recommended that increasing fibre in the diet helps to prevent constipation. But it has also been found that this can cause constipation to worsen in some people. Generally it makes sense to encourage the client to eat a range of foods and include fruit and vegetables and some cereals and pulses (peas and beans). As with many things, some foods (such as prunes) seem to work well in preventing constipation for some people and not for others and it is important to find out what the client finds effective. If bran is being added to food (to increase its fibre content) it is very important that the client drinks plenty of liquid (the bran absorbs liquid) to prevent constipation occurring.

Eating a range of foods requires a working set of teeth

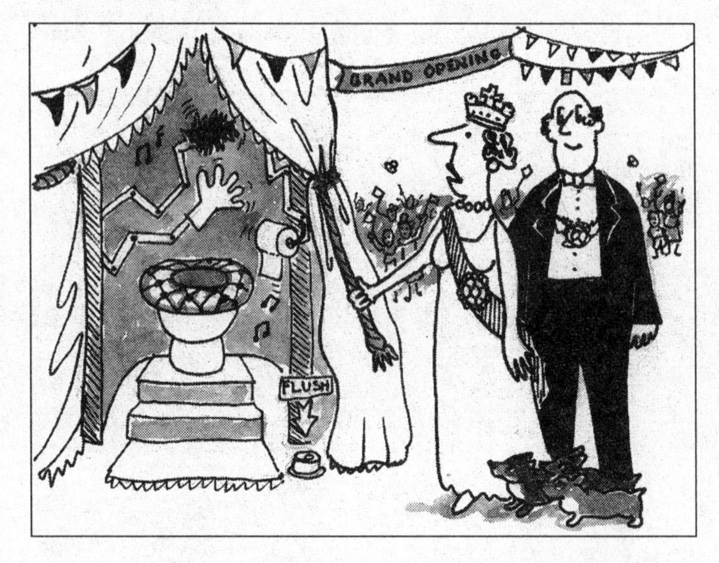

and a pain-free mouth. Ensure that any dental problems are dealt with and sore mouths or gums are reported.

General surroundings

The surroundings that the client lives in (and you work in) also play a part in helping or hindering continence. Toilet signs need to be very bold so that they can be clearly seen from a distance. To help clients who are confused or who have problems with memory or sight, toilets may be indicated by **clear** symbols or a picture of a toilet, rather than a written word, or all toilet doors may be painted one colour.

Look at where the client likes to spend her time and the distance she needs to travel, together with the obstacles she needs to pass, in order to get to the toilet. Beds and chairs should be at the correct height for the individual to be able to get out of easily. Heavy doors can prevent easy access to the toilet, as can slippery floors, loose mats, stairs or the sheer distance. Improving access to existing toilets can help prevent incontinence. Better still might be the provision of more "user-friendly" toilets.

Reality orientation

Keeping clients in touch with reality can also play a part in helping them to stay continent. Residential care can seem a strange and muddling place, particularly to a slightly confused person. It can be difficult for the client to remember where she is, what time of day it is or who the different people are and what they do. You can help clients to stay in better contact with reality by including information about the time, the people and the place in general conversation.

When talking to the client gently remind her of the time: ("It's 5 o'clock in the afternoon Mrs. Jenkins, would you like to go to the toilet?"). Use the client's name (but find out first how she likes to be addressed) and avoid using words like Dearie or Pet, as these words don't help the client remember who they are and can be offensive.

Mention where you are and who you are when talking: ("Hello, Mrs Bridges, my name is Elaine and I work in the home. We are in the sitting room now; when you want to use the toilet remember that the toilet door is green. The nearest toilet is just opposite the door to the sitting room.")

Clocks and calendars can help failing memories and personal mementos of family and friends, such as photos at the bedside, can help to remind the client who she is. Often clients with poor short term memories can remember things from a long time ago. Engaging clients in conversations about themselves and things that interest them and are enjoyable is as important as assisting with their physical care. Keeping people as occupied, stimulated and motivated as possible helps clients to maintain an interest in themselves and their surroundings and reduces the risk of incontinence.

Helping clients to stay continent involves a whole package of activities and cannot be separated from the client's care as a whole. Be positive, and with your help many clients will be able to stay continent.

KEY POINTS

- Clients who have recently been admitted to a home or hospital are likely to be particularly at risk of being incontinent.
- Good toileting practices, good toilet facilities and toilet alternatives can help to prevent incontinence.
- Clients should be taken to the toilet at times that suit them rather than at routine times.
- Be sensitive about toileting and try to increase privacy and reduce the client's embarrassment.
- Clothing adaptations may make toileting quicker and easier.
- Clients need to drink at least 1-2 litres every day, but the timing of drinking can be adjusted to help reduce incontinence.
- Toilet signs should be bold. Distance and obstacles to the toilet should be reduced.
- Reality orientation may help to keep confused clients in touch with daily life, which can help them stay continent.

3

Why does incontinence happen?

How the bladder and bowel work and what can go wrong. What else affects continence – medicines, urine infection, constipation, mobility, communication, confusion, depression, getting older. Routines and habits. Just laziness?

Staying continent is not always possible. Sometimes the bladder or bowel does not work properly, or there are other physical or mental problems that cause incontinence. Often, particularly for elderly or disabled people, it is a combination of problems that is to blame.

Why do we have a bladder and how does the bladder work?

If we didn't have a bladder we would be wet all the time. The kidneys are constantly producing urine (which contains waste chemicals and water from the body) rather like a dripping tap (Fig 3.1). The job of the bladder is to collect and store the urine and then to empty by pushing

The bladder needs to:

- be able to store and hold urine
- have a good seal at the outlet.
- be able to empty completely.

the urine out when it becomes rather full.

Storing and holding urine

The bladder is a bag made of muscle and can stretch while it is being filled with urine. The normal bladder capacity (the amount it can hold comfortably) is about 400-600 ml (about a pint).

Obviously it would be very inconvenient if the bladder emptied when we weren't expecting it (and this is exactly what happens to some people who are incontinent), so the bladder is controlled by nerves from the brain and spinal cord.

When the bladder is getting full (about 250ml/half a pint/two cups or more) messages are sent from the bladder to the brain, so that we know that we need to "go". We can then send messages back to the bladder and put off emptying the bladder for a while. In this way the bladder is able to continue to store urine until it is comfortably full and a toilet is accessible.

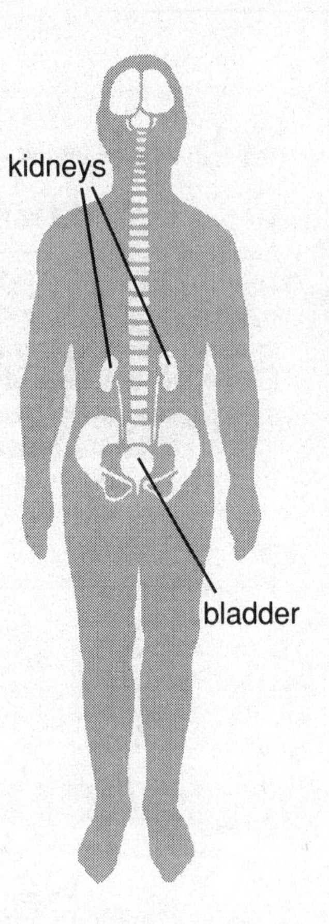

Fig 3.1 Position of bladder and kidneys in the body.

Keeping the bladder outlet sealed

The bladder stores the urine **above** the tube that allows the urine out (the urethra or bladder outlet) so we need to have some way of stopping the urine from leaking. Imagine the bladder as being a bit like a balloon filled with water, with the outlet at the bottom. If you didn't hold the balloon outlet together between finger and thumb the water would come dribbling out. To stop any leaking the body has its own "finger and thumb" in the form of a ring of muscles called a sphincter. While the bladder is storing urine the muscles are closed shut so that urine cannot leak out. When we pass urine the muscles relax and allow urine out.

The sphincter muscle is helped by a "sling" of muscles called the "pelvic floor". These muscles are attached to the bone at the bottom of the spine (the coccyx) and run between the legs to the bone at the front (the pubic bone). The body passages, the urethra, vagina and anus (exit from the bowel) pass through this muscle (Fig 3.2).

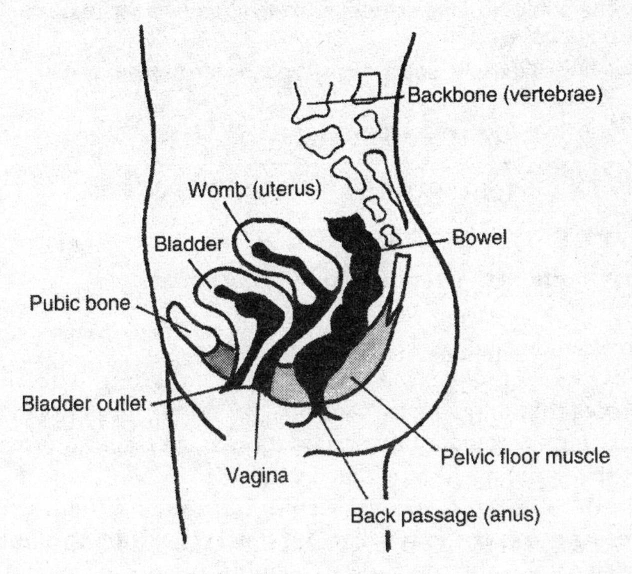

Fig 3.2 Female side view shows pelvic floor and body passages.

Emptying the bladder

Finally, having collected and stored a few cupfulls of urine the bladder needs to be able to "push out" the urine. When we have decided where and when we want to pass urine messages are sent from the brain to the bladder to make the bladder **push out** the urine. The urine then passes through the urethra and out of the body.

The frequency of bladder emptying varies from person to person. We all know people who seem to pass urine very often, perhaps about 8-10 times in 24 hours, whilst others seem to be able to last for hours without doing so. The number of times an "average" person passes urine ranges from about 4-7 times a day.

- The bladder holds about 400-600ml when comfortably full.
- The bladder is made of muscle and controlled by nerves.
- The purpose of the bladder is to store urine and then push urine out.
- A ring of muscle (sphincter) surrounds the bladder outlet (urethra).
- The "average" person passes urine 4-7 times per day.

What can go wrong with the bladder?

Urge incontinence -
problems with storing and holding urine

Urge incontinence is caused by an over-active bladder. This happens because something goes wrong with the nerves that allow us to "put off" passing urine; the bladder starts to push out urine as soon as messages are sent to the spine and brain that we need to "go". The result is a strong **urge** to pass urine and great difficulty in **holding on**. If the toilet is not reached within a minute or two (or sometimes even seconds) then incontinence will result. You probably know clients who call for the

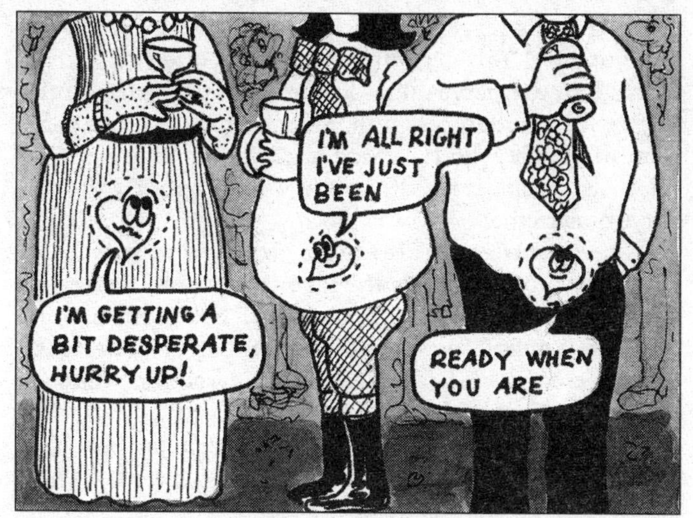

The bladder sends messages to the brain when it is getting full.

toilet urgently, but then have already been incontinent by the time you have brought the commode or taken them to the toilet. **Urge** incontinence may well be the problem.

You may occasionally have felt a similar experience yourself. If you want to pass urine, go and find a toilet, but then discover that it is occupied you may find that you are dancing up and down outside "dying" to go to the toilet. This is because your bladder is getting ready to pass urine (it thinks you should be sitting on the toilet by now) and starts to push, giving you a strong "urge".

However, people with urge incontinence experience this problem several times a day and may well have to pass urine during the night or possibly wet the bed. Often the urge to pass urine occurs when the bladder is only partly full of urine so the person ends up passing frequent, small amounts of urine.

Urge problems do not always result in incontinence.

If the toilet is reached quickly enough there may be no incontinence. But urge incontinence is often caused by damage to the nerves that also affects other parts of the body. So, for example, urge incontinence is quite common in people who have had a stroke, or have multiple sclerosis, Parkinson's disease or other disorders of the nervous system.

These diseases can also cause problems with mobility (the person **can't reach** the toilet easily) and finger and hand movements (it is difficult to pull down pants, open flies, or lift clothing up). So a number of continence actions are affected (see chapter 2). Urge incontinence has been found to be the most common bladder problem affecting people in residential settings, probably because many clients have disorders of the nervous system like those mentioned above.

Stress incontinence -

problems with keeping the bladder outlet sealed

Activities such as coughing, laughing, sneezing or even just walking, put pressure on the bladder. If the **pelvic floor** or sphincter muscles are weakened (usually by childbirth) so that the bladder outlet is not properly sealed, then it may be impossible for the sphincter to stand the extra pressure. Think of the water-filled balloon again: if you pressed down sharply on the balloon with your hand and you weren't holding the outlet tightly between finger and thumb, a jet of water would leak out.

In **stress** incontinence urine leaks out without any feeling that you need to pass urine. Usually the amount of urine is small, but enough to cause discomfort and wet patches on clothes.

After the change of life women's **hormones** fall and the vagina, urethra and surrounding area can become sore and dry. This may result in the urethra not closing properly and can contribute to stress incontinence.

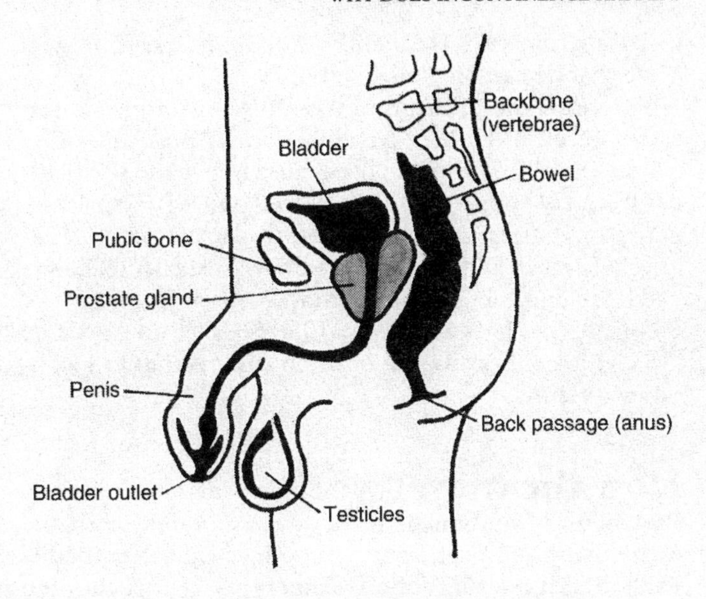

Fig 3.3 Side view of male showing enlarged prostate gland.

Stress incontinence mostly affects women but can occur in men after a **prostate** operation.

Overflow incontinence -

problems with emptying the bladder

In some people the bladder may become "over-filled" with urine because it is unable to empty properly. This can be caused by two different problems.

Firstly, an **obstruction** (usually an enlarged prostate gland in men, Fig 3.3) may prevent urine from passing out of the urethra even though the person is trying to pass urine. Imagine squeezing the water filled balloon (as if you were "pushing" the water out) with one hand, but with your finger and thumb held very tightly round the outlet, very little water would come out. Because the bladder is constantly full of urine the person may want to pass urine very frequently, but finds when he gets there that he can only pass a dribble.

Secondly, the problem of **overflow** incontinence can occur because the bladder muscle can't push the urine out properly. This is usually because **nerves** to the bladder from the spinal cord have been damaged, (usually by injury or disease, such as diabetes), so that the bladder muscle is weak and floppy like an over-stretched balloon.

The main problem with both the causes of this type of incontinence is that the bladder doesn't empty. The bladder is continually full of urine and overflows; incontinence results.

How the bowel works

Part of the function of the bowel is to deal with the waste that is left over from the food we eat. After food is swallowed it goes into the **stomach** where it is churned up into a "watery mash". The stomach then pushes the mash into the bowel which is rather like a hosepipe coiled inside our abdomen (tummy). The bowel is made up of two parts: small and large. The **small bowel** absorbs the nutritional part of food (protein, vitamins etc) and the **large bowel** removes water from the left over waste food matter to form faeces.

The last part of the large intestine is called the **rectum** (Figs 3.2 & 3.3) and this ends in a ring of muscle, forming a sphincter called the anus. When sufficient faeces enter the rectum, nerves send messages from the rectum to the brain giving the feeling that we need to empty the bowel. If it is not convenient, we can delay passing faeces and the sensation will eventually go away. When it is convenient messages are sent from the brain to the rectum; the anal sphincter muscles relax, the rectal muscle pushes faeces out. This action is usually assisted by "pushing down" using the abdominal (tummy) muscles.

As with the bladder there is variation from person to

person in the frequency of bowel actions. As many as three times a day to as little as once every three days is considered "normal". A normal bowel motion should be formed in a lump, soft and easy to pass.

What can go wrong with the bowel

In elderly people by far the most common cause of faecal incontinence is severe **constipation** or faecal impaction. The rectum becomes filled with a large mass of faeces, which may be soft or hard. Faecal incontinence may occur because the anal sphincter relaxes and some faeces are passed before the person feels the need to "go". The person may still have normal bowel actions, but does not manage to clear the bowel of the mass, so incontinence can still occur. Sometimes the faecal impaction can cause liquid faeces to escape through the anus around the faecal impaction. In this case it seems as if the person is having diarrhoea, but constipation is the real problem.

As with the bladder, problems with the **nervous system** can affect the proper functioning of the bowel. There may be loss of ability to feel the need to pass faeces, the ability to put off passing faeces and also the ability to push down to empty the bowel. So faeces may be passed without the person knowing. Lack of sensation and inability to push also results in constipation.

It is also worth remembering that a sudden episode of diarrhoea may make anyone incontinent, particularly if there are problems reaching the toilet.

What else can affect continence?

Medicines

Many medicines affect the bladder and bowel in some way. **Diuretics** (water tablets) cause the kidneys to produce a larger amount of urine than usual. This puts a strain on continence because the bladder is often filled very quickly, which results in the client wanting to pass urine frequently and urgently.

Problems with **holding on** and **reaching** the toilet often result. If there already is an underlying urge problem then incontinence is very likely.

Medicines that cause drowsiness can affect continence. **Sedation** (sleeping tablets) may mean that the client sleeps through messages from the bladder that urine needs to be passed. Unfortunately a good night's sleep may then mean a wet bed.

The ability of the bladder to empty properly may also be affected by certain medicines and this can lead to overflow incontinence. These include tablets for:

lowering blood pressure	eg propranolol;
breathing	eg salbutamol
Parkinson's disease	eg levodopa
depression	eg amitriptyline
mental illness	eg chlorpromazine.

Constipation is a side-effect of many medicines and this can lead to urinary incontinence (see below) or faecal incontinence. Tablets or liquids containing codeine (such as some pain killers and cough linctus), some blood pressure lowering tablets, and some tablets used in the treatment of urinary incontinence are just a few examples of constipating medicines.

Other medicines may have side effects on the bladder. If a continent person becomes incontinent shortly after a new medicine has been prescribed this should be reported; the problem may be related to the medicine.

Bladder infection

Anybody who has had cystitis knows the trouble that a bladder infection can cause. A urine infection can make the bladder very irritated and urine is passed frequently and with urgency (and often pain). Clients with problems reaching the toilet may well become incontinent, although usually this will be temporary.

People who have problems emptying the bladder (for example in overflow incontinence) may have urine infections most of the time; but these infections are less likely to cause the same urgency problems and do not necessarily cause incontinence.

Constipation

If the bowel becomes very full with packed faeces then this bulky mass may press on the bladder. This may make an urge incontinence problem worse by irritating the bladder or may press on the urethra and lead to overflow incontinence (Fig 3.4 shows how constipation can affect the bladder outflow). Either way it is also likely to make the client feel unwell, possibly **confused** and also very much at risk of faecal incontinence.

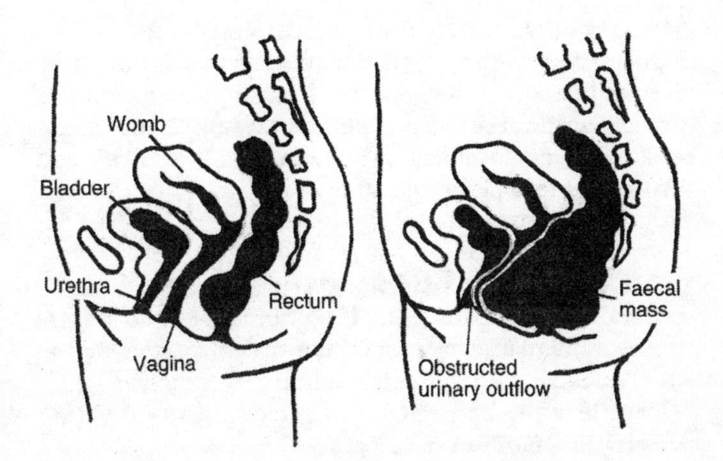

Fig 3.4 Side view of female showing how constipation can affect the bladder outflow and cause incontinence of urine.

Mobility

Getting to the toilet or getting the toilet to you is crucial for continence. A completely mobile person may be able to keep continent despite quite a severe bladder problem, while a very immobile person may become incontinent with a much milder problem, just because they have difficulties reaching the toilet.

Most people in residential homes or long stay wards have mobility problems of some kind or another.

Hands and fingers

Arthritic, shaky or weak hands and fingers mean that removing clothes and using aids such as urinals can be very difficult. Hand and finger problems often contribute to the "slowness" of toileting which can so easily tip the balance from continence to incontinence

Seeing, hearing and speaking

Sight problems can mean that the client cannot easily identify the toilet (or get there easily) and of course hearing and speaking problems may make the whole business of communicating toileting needs difficult and demanding for clients and staff.

Confusion and dementia

Infections, problems with lungs or heart and severe stress can all cause temporary confusion, particularly in elderly people, and this can result in incontinence.

People with dementia may become incontinent because they no longer recognise the need to pass urine or may not be able to identify that a toilet is the place where they should "go". But many people with severe dementia remain continent, probably because of their lifelong toileting habits. If you have spent 70 years or more passing urine when sitting on the toilet with your pants down, then for many people this will continue automatically; even though many other brain functions seem to have been lost. Dementia does not necessarily result in incontinence and it is important that other causes of incontinence are not overlooked.

Depression

People who are depressed often neglect themselves, including their personal appearance and body functions. Depression may well go undetected, particularly in someone with communication problems or in clients who have always "kept themselves to themselves".

Mental problems and brain injury

People with disorders of their nervous system may experience mental problems that can contribute to incontinence. Loss of motivation, inhibitions and concentration, as well as depression can all occur as a result of damage to the nervous system resulting from disorders such as stroke, Parkinson's disease and multiple sclerosis.

Getting older

Most elderly people are not incontinent, but incontinence becomes more common as we get older. These are some of the main reasons why:

- More urine tends to be produced, especially at night (the kidneys work less effectively).
- Urine infections are more common.
- All bladder problems (urge, stress, and overflow) are more common.

- In women the urethra may not close so well due to hormone changes.
- In men the prostate gland often becomes larger.
- More medicines are prescribed for elderly people.
- Constipation is more common.
- Mobility and other physical and mental problems are more likely.

Routines and habits

Personal toileting routines and habits may be disrupted by the routines of the home or hospital (see chapter 2) and cause incontinence. It is also possible that the way incontinence is dealt with may make incontinence rewarding, particularly for people with dementia. Being washed and having pads changed may come with a smile, a chat and a touch from the care assistant. This may be the client's only source of such physical and social contact, especially when staff levels are low. There may seem to be nothing to gain in staying dry or using the toilet independently (see chapter 5 for ideas on how to reward continence).

Temporary incontinence

Incontinence may occur temporarily as a result of an illness, such as a chest infection or a flare-up of an old problem such as arthritis. Any problem that suddenly reduces mobility, eating and drinking, mental functioning, or interferes with any continence actions can lead to temporary incontinence. But expect the incontinence to improve as the client gets better and in the meantime pay close attention to ways of helping the client to stay continent (see chapter 2).

Just laziness?

It is often tempting to think that "laziness" is the cause of an incontinence problem. Some clients may seem to take little notice of their toileting needs, may appear unconcerned about their incontinence or seem generally unmotivated and indifferent. Some clients may also be continent at times and not at others, seeming to indicate that they could control their bladder or bowel if they tried.

But the problem with putting incontinence down to laziness is that it puts the "blame" on the client and stops staff looking for other causes of the incontinence. Considering the large number of things that are known to cause incontinence, it is very unlikely that no other cause but laziness would be found.

It is also worth remembering that people with nervous system disorders, particularly multiple sclerosis and Parkinson's disease, have problems that vary from day to day. There are times when they can do things and times when they can't. Tiredness is also a common problem with some of these disorders and clients may find the effort of toileting is too much on some days. This is the nature of their disease, not "just laziness" as it may well appear. Similarly, problems with motivation and apathy may well be a result of the client's disease or disorder.

A number of causes

For many people, incontinence is not just caused by one thing, but by a number of causes, which together prevent a person from successfully carrying out the actions necessary for continence.

KEY POINTS

- The bladder is made of muscle and controlled by nerves.
- The bladder stores and holds urine, keeps urine sealed in and pushes urine out when it becomes full.
- Urge incontinence is caused by an over-active bladder. This means that the bladder cannot store or hold much urine.
- Stress incontinence is caused by weak sphincter muscles. This means that the bladder outlet is not well sealed and can leak.
- Overflow incontinence may be caused by an obstruction to the bladder outlet which prevents the bladder from emptying completely.
- Overflow incontinence may also be caused by damage to the bladder nerves. The bladder is then unable to push the urine out properly.
- Constipation is the most common cause of faecal incontinence.
- Medicines, urine infections and constipation can all contribute to urinary incontinence.
- Problems with mobility, hands and fingers, communication and confusion and dementia may lead to incontinence.
- Brain injury and depression may affect motivation and cause people to neglect their body functions.
- As the bladder and kidneys get older changes occur that make incontinence more likely.
- Laziness is rarely the cause of incontinence.

4
Finding out why

A team approach. Assessment information, examinations and tests. Finding out how much and how often. Keeping a chart.

If you had a pain in your chest, you would probably go along to your doctor expecting them to find the cause of the problem. Is it indigestion, a chest infection or a heart problem? The cause will need to be found so that the correct treatment can be given. Indigestion tablets won't help a chest infection much. In just the same way the cause or causes of incontinence described in chapter 3 will need to be found.

Different bladder or bowel problems have different treatments; clients will have different mental and physical problems that may be part of their incontinence problem. Some causes may be obvious but others are more difficult to find. Making an assessment to try to find out why a client is incontinent is essential so that the right methods can be used to help improve the problem and sometimes cure it.

A team approach

As a member of the team you will play an important part in helping to find out why a client is incontinent. But other people with different skills and expertise will also need to be involved. Ideally the client will be assessed by a nurse who has skills in improving continence problems. The client's doctor may also need to be involved; certain medicines may need to be prescribed

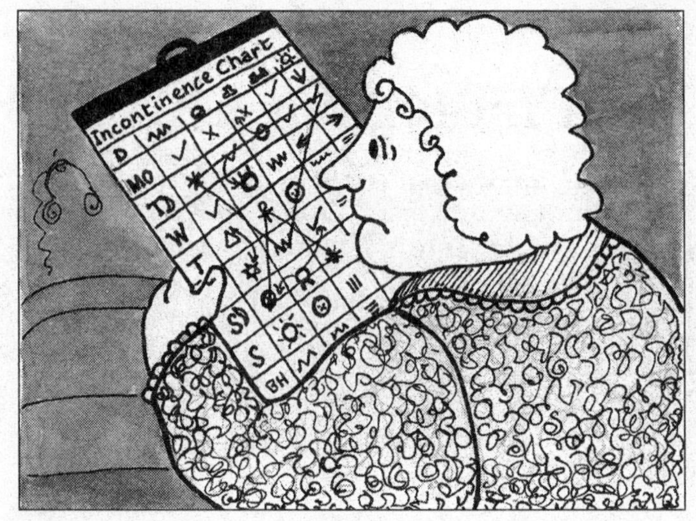

Keep a chart, but keep it simple

(see chapter 5) and tests and investigations may need to be organised. The doctor may also refer the client to a hospital specialist such as a urologist or gynaecologist.

A continence advisor may also help. Continence advisors are usually nurses who have had special training in continence management. They give advice to incontinent people and to carers and may also give teaching sessions about incontinence. One may be available in your area. The Incontinence Information Helpline (see appendix, page 89) will tell you your nearest advisor. Other health care professionals such as a physiotherapist or occupational therapist are also likely to be involved if the client could benefit from their skills and advice.

Assessment information, examinations and tests

Talking and **listening** to the client is usually the best place to start, but remember that people use different words for passing urine and faeces (see Glossary). The way the client describes her incontinence problem can often help to indicate which type of bladder problem she has. For example, a client with an **urge** type bladder problem may say that she always has to rush to the toilet and cannot hold on for long enough to get there. The nurse or continence advisor will usually therefore take a detailed **history** of the incontinence problem from the client. Talking to the client also helps to provide background information such as how the client feels about the problem, how it is affecting her life, how much liquid she is drinking, what aids she is using and whether or not they work well.

The person doing the **assessment** needs to gain the client's **confidence** and **trust** at this stage. Sometimes the client may want someone who knows them well (such as yourself) to help in the discussion. The client will also need information herself; it is important that she understands what is happening throughout the assessment and has an opportunity to make her own decisions about whether or not she is willing for any aspect of the assessment (or treatment) to go ahead.

Obviously it is not always possible to obtain so much detail from the client. Brain damage, confusion, dementia, severe depression and communication problems may all mean that only a limited amount of information (sometimes none) is available from the client. Medical and nursing notes, members of the health care team (you for example), and relatives may then be the main source of information.

Observation of toileting can provide vital information about the client's problems with communication, mobility, hands and fingers and the use or need for toileting aids. As it is usually care assistants who have the greatest knowledge about problems with toileting, you will need to pass on this information to the person doing the assessment. It may be useful to use the headings under toileting in chapter 2 to describe the client's abilities and problems fully.

A physical examination should be carried out by the nurse or doctor to check for problems and possible causes of incontinence. For example, a rectal examination may be done to find out the size of a man's prostate gland (which can be felt with a finger from inside the rectum) or to find out if there is a problem with constipation. A woman may be examined vaginally for signs of hormone shortage or to assess the the muscles of the pelvic floor (see chapter 3).

Medicines that the client is taking need to be checked to ensure that they are not contributing to incontinence.

A urine specimen may need to be tested to see if there is infection present.

A catheter (a hollow tube) may be passed into the bladder after the client has passed urine, to measure the amount of urine left, this is called the "residual urine". A large amount (above 100ml) may indicate overflow incontinence.

Urodynamic studies may be organised for the client. This test is usually carried out in a hospital outpatient department and is the most accurate method of diagnosing bladder problems.

It does however require complete cooperation from the client as it involves having tubes passed into the bladder and rectum. These studies are usually only for people who may be going to have an operation, people with complex bladder problems or who have bladder problems that have not shown improvement with the usual treatments.

Finding out how much and how often

Assessment of incontinence may include:
- **Talking** and taking a history
- **Toileting** observation
- **Physical** examination
- **Sending** a specimen of urine to the laboratory for testing
- **Measuring** residual urine
- **Urodynamic** studies
- **Keeping** a chart

It is one thing to **know** that a client has an incontinence problem, but quite another thing to know how often it is occurring. Think for a minute and try to work out how often you passed urine yesterday and the day before.

You probably came up with a rough idea of the number of times you passed urine, but possibly not very easily. It is even more difficult to estimate the number of times a client passes urine or is incontinent.

Doing different shifts and caring for a number of clients at a time means that a guess is often the best that can be done. The frequency of incontinence may also vary from day to day for various reasons; for example it may be that some care assistants are better at toileting than others or that the client was particularly constipated at that time.

Finding out how much and how often is important because this information provides the **baseline** for the client. Most incontinence is not cured overnight and it is hard to spot any gradual improvement if you don't know how often the problem was occurring in the first place.

The best way to find out how much and how often is to keep a chart. Charts may be made up from blank paper, or printed charts are available from a number of different companies who produce continence products (eg Molnlycke, Coloplast). A common example of a simple chart is shown in Fig 4.1.

TIME	MON		TUES		WED		THURS		FRI		SAT		SUN	
6am														
7am														
8am														
9am														
10am														
11am														
12am														
1pm														
2pm														
3pm														
4pm														
5pm														
6pm														
7pm														
8pm														
9pm														
10pm														
11pm														
12pm														
1am														
2am														
3am														
4am														
5am														
TOTAL														

Please tick in this column every time you use the toilet. ☐

Please tick in this column every time you are wet. ▒

Fig 4.1 A simple chart.

Keeping a chart

If possible the client should keep the chart herself. This involves the client closely in the assessment (which has been found to be helpful). The client records with a tick in one column (on the right day and time) when she passes urine in the toilet and a tick in another column when she is incontinent of urine. But charts can be tricky to fill in and you may need to help her. For this reason try and keep the chart as simple as possible.

Clients who need to be reminded to use the toilet or who need to be toileted will often need to have more information recorded on the chart and may well not be able to keep a chart themselves. In particular it is useful to record if the client did not pass urine in the toilet when she was taken there. There is space for special instructions on most charts and a cross may be used to indicate that the client was taken to the toilet but did not use it. To ensure privacy remember to keep the chart out of public view.

One of the difficulties of keeping a chart is that you may only know that a client has been incontinent of urine when she is actually taken to the toilet and the pad is found to be wet. Checking the pad (discreetly) hourly or two hourly and recording what you find (eg 0 for dry pad) helps to pinpoint more accurately when incontinence is happening. Incontinence pads with wetness indicators are particularly useful for this, as it is possible to see if the pad is wet with the minimum of trouble for the client, and without feeling the pad.

Some charts have been designed to record all the above information and you may find these to be better than "customising" the simple charts. An example of such a chart is shown in Fig 4.2. This chart also allows for marking roughly how much urine is lost when incontinent and how much urine is passed on the toilet. There is also room for comments: it may be that certain events (such as visitors) are associated with incontinence or that the incontinence only happens in certain places (such as in the dayroom).

Whichever method is chosen, keep the chart for about 5-7 days to provide the baseline. Then take a good look at the chart: it may indicate a **pattern** of incontinence.

Date TIME	BLADDER Incontinent of urine	DRY	Voided correctly	BOWEL Incontinent	Normal	Comments
6am	◊ ◊	○	◇ ml			
7am	◊ ◊	○	◇ ml			
8am	◊ ◊	○	◇ ml			
9am	◊ ◊	○	◇ ml			
10am	◊ ◊	○	◇ ml			
11am	◊ ◊	○	◇ ml			
12am	◊ ◊	○	◇ ml			
1pm	◊ ◊	○	◇ ml			
2pm	◊ ◊	○	◇ ml			
3pm	◊ ◊	○	◇ ml			
4pm	◊ ◊	○	◇ ml			
5pm	◊ ◊	○	◇ ml			
6pm	◊ ◊	○	◇ ml			
7pm	◊ ◊	○	◇ ml			
8pm	◊ ◊	○	◇ ml			
9pm	◊ ◊	○	◇ ml			
10pm	◊ ◊	○	◇ ml			
11pm	◊ ◊	○	◇ ml			
12pm	◊ ◊	○	◇ ml			
1am	◊ ◊	○	◇ ml			
2am	◊ ◊	○	◇ ml			
3am	◊ ◊	○	◇ ml			
4am	◊ ◊	○	◇ ml			
5am	◊ ◊	○	◇ ml			
TOTAL						

Cross correct symbol at the hour closest to to the time patient is checked.

Incontinent, small amount. Dry.

Incontinent, large amount. Voided correctly.

Fig 4.2 A more detailed chart.

For example, the client may always be incontinent in the mornings after taking a water tablet (diuretic). A chart is also useful for indicating what type of bladder problem is present: passing small, frequent amounts of urine may indicate urge or (possibly overflow) incontinence.

A full assessment should enable a picture to be built up of all the problems that are causing the client's incontinence.

KEY POINTS

- Assessment of incontinence is vital to find out why the client is incontinent.
- A nurse or continence advisor will usually assess the client.
- Information from care assistants and other members of the team need to be included in the assessment.
- Assessment may involve the following:

  Talking to the client

  Checking and treating any constipation

  Checking urine for infection

  Keeping a chart for 4 -7 days

  Observing toileting and noting problems

  Checking medicines prescribed

  Physical examination

  Measurement of residual urine and/or urodynamic studies

5
What can be done?

Focusing on the resident. Dealing with constipation. Dealing with infection. Treatments for bladder problems. Providing an individualised toileting programme. Rewards and encouragement. Combining ways to improve incontinence.

If you have followed the guidelines set out so far, you will have done a great deal already. Using the general principles of "staying continent" and understanding why incontinence happens can make a great difference in helping to keep people continent in residential care, and will also help people who are already incontinent.

This chapter will focus on different methods that can be used to improve incontinence. "Finding out why" a client is incontinent will often lead to a number of possible **causes** being uncovered. There is often a **bladder** or **bowel problem** underlying the incontinence together with a number of other problems, some more open to improvement than others.

How can you make a difference?

Doing something about incontinence often involves tackling many problems. Making small differences to several problems may well be more possible than "curing" one problem, and may help to tip the balance away from incontinence.

But remember that continence will not be possible for all clients. Don't be disappointed if your efforts do not help a client; others are sure to benefit.

Focusing on the client

Any change in care or new treatment that is offered needs to be talked over with the client first. A lot of people know very little about how their bladder and bowels work and need a clear explanation of their problems and how they may be helped. The client is then free to make a choice about treatment and changes in care. Gaining cooperation and positive involvement from the client is not only an important principle but is also essential for many of the methods used to improve incontinence.

It is also vital to ensure that client care is consistent. When planning how to improve continence all staff (senior nurses/managers, day and night staff) should work together and follow the care planned for the client.

Dealing with constipation

It may seem a bit odd to start this section by looking at the problem of constipation, but this problem is usually the cause of faecal incontinence and will make any bladder problem worse. There is little point in doing anything before dealing with constipation.

If **faecal impaction** is present then usually the best way to treat it is to give an enema (usually phosphate or a microenema) every other day until the mass has cleared. Occasionally a nurse may need to remove the faeces manually, particularly if they are very hard.

Once the impaction has been removed it is important to pay attention to preventing constipation and keeping the bowel clear. Looking at the client's food and drink intake, improving mobility (see "eating and drinking" and "staying mobile", chapter 2) and checking medicines to make sure that they are not causing incontinence are the best ways of preventing constipation, but regular laxatives may also be necessary.

Some clients with disorders of the nervous system

may rarely be able to pass faeces themselves and may need an enema two (or sometimes three) times a week to clear the bowel. A similar "planned bowel action" scheme may also be useful for elderly clients with dementia, if constipation followed by impaction and faecal incontinence is a continuous problem.

Dealing with infection

An acute urine infection with symptoms (such as pain, urgency, fever etc) will need treatment from a doctor. Any urine infection may be a sign that the client is not able to empty the bladder properly and may therefore have overflow incontinence. The management for this is described later in the chapter.

How can bladder problems be treated?

Urge incontinence -

bladder training and medicines

Clients with urge incontinence usually feel the need to pass urine suddenly and urgently; if the person does not reach the toilet (or the toilet facility does not reach her) in time then incontinence occurs. Because the urge to pass urine tends to occur before the bladder has much urine inside she passes urine very frequently. Fear of being incontinent also means that urine may be passed before there is any real need.

Keeping a chart usually shows a pattern of **frequency** (having to pass urine every two hours or more) and incontinence. A typical chart from someone with this problem is shown in Appendix IV, page 93.

Bladder training is probably the best treatment for urge incontinence, but is not suitable for all clients. Those who are able to complete charts themselves and are able to understand and cooperate with the training programme are likely to be most successful.

The aim of bladder training is to prevent incontinence and to reduce the problems of frequency and urgency so that the client has a more normal pattern of toilet visits.

Once the **baseline** chart has been completed (see chapter 4) the client is asked to **hang on** between visits to the toilet for longer than she normally does. So, for example, if the client is passing urine about every hour and a half on the baseline chart, the she is asked to try and hang on for perhaps two hours between toilet visits. Incontinence often occurs whilst the person is desperately trying to get to the toilet, so the client may find it helpful to try and sit quietly and concentrate on trying to control the bladder; counting slowly may be useful. After a while the bladder stops trying to push the urine out and the urge goes away.

Once the client is able to hang on for the time stated (two hours in this case) which usually takes a week or two, then she is asked to aim for a longer time (two and a half hours). The times between visits to the toilet are gradually increased until the client can hang on for about three to four hours. Usually no times are set for the night time and passing urine frequently at night or bedwetting gets better along with the daytime.

The person may need to pass urine more often at some times during the day than others, such as in the morning after a water tablet, so it is important to adjust the times to suit the client, perhaps aiming for every two hours in the morning and every two and a half hours in the afternoon.

It isn't easy to do bladder training and most people need plenty of encouragement. It's a bit like giving up smoking: the longing to give in can be very strong! Bladder training works best when the times that the client is aiming for are possible; gradual improvement is much better than risking failure by expecting too much. If the client doesn't wear a pad it may be a good idea to use a small pad while doing bladder training to help with security and confidence.

Some medicines can decrease the problem of urge incontinence by reducing the ability of the bladder to "push out" the urine. The most common tablet used for this is **oxybutynin**. This may be prescribed for clients who have urge incontinence but are unable to take part in a bladder training programme. Oxybutynin may also be prescribed for clients who can undertake bladder training, as it may help to make the programme quicker and more successful. But like many medicines, oxybutynin has some unwanted side effects such as double vision, dry mouth and constipation and these are sometimes very troublesome.

Constipation, in particular, should be expected and action taken to prevent it if a client is taking oxybutynin (see above and chapter 2).

For most people with urge incontinence the problem will improve or disappear altogether with the above treatment. But for some people it is never possible to put off passing urine for long and some urgency still remains. Quick access to the toilet is then a priority, and alternatives to the toilet and toileting aids may be needed (see chapter 2).

Stress incontinence -

pelvic floor exercises and hormone therapy

Stress incontinence usually occurs because the ring of muscle surrounding the urethra has become weak and is unable to prevent urine **leaking out** when there is **extra pressure** on the bladder, such as when you cough or laugh. This ring of muscle is surrounded by the muscles of the pelvic floor (see chapter 3) and it is often possible to strengthen these muscles with exercises (pp.93-94) so that the sphincter muscle becomes stronger and less likely to allow any leaking.

Learning how to do these exercises takes time and the client must be able to understand and take part fully. Nobody can exercise these muscles for anyone else! As with the treatment for urge incontinence it is vital to be aware of the progress of any client doing pelvic floor exercises and to give her encouragement to help her continue. Learning these exercises is also useful for people with urge incontinence as they can be helpful for learning to hang on.

Another method of doing pelvic floor exercises involves the use of **cones** (Fig 5.1). A cone is inserted into the vagina and the muscles of the pelvic floor automatically tighten to prevent the cone from falling out. The cone is usually kept in for about 10 minutes at a time while the client is walking about (not sitting down). When the cone can be kept in easily a heavier cone is used instead. Cones come in sets of three or four.

Being able to exercise the pelvic floor is an important skill for any woman. Stress incontinence is such a common problem that as many as half of women may be affected at some time in their lives. Learning pelvic floor exercises helps to **prevent** the problem of stress incontinence; if you are a woman you may wish to learn the exercises yourself.

Women who have problems with a sore, dry vagina (and urethra) after the change of life may benefit from hormone therapy. This can help to reduce stress incontinence if the dryness results in the urethra not closing properly.

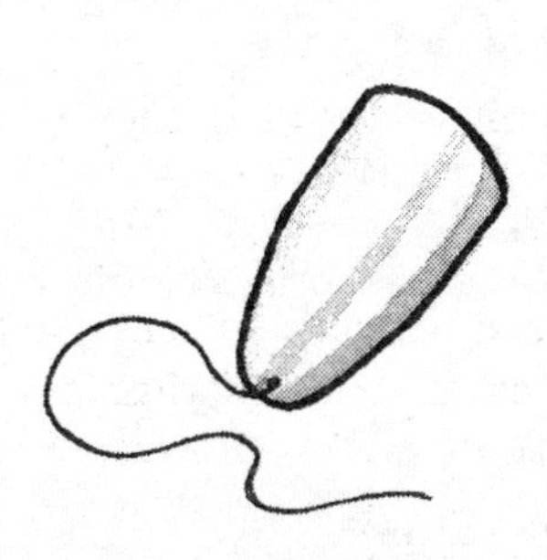

Fig 5.1 Cone for pelvic floor exercises.

Sometimes an operation is required to improve stress incontinence, usually for women who have already done pelvic floor exercises but are still incontinent.

Overflow incontinence –

intermittent catheterisation and surgery

If the bladder is unable to empty properly overflow incontinence can result. If this is because of medicines or constipation then these will need to be dealt with first. **Intermittent catheterisation** is an effective treatment if the overflow incontinence is caused by the bladder being unable to push the urine out. The urine in the bladder is removed by passing a hollow tube (catheter) through the urethra and into the bladder. The urine drains out and the catheter is **removed** (Fig 5.2). This is different from an ordinary catheter which is left in the bladder and attached to a bag (see chapter 6). Sometimes it is only necessary for a catheter to be passed once a day or even as little as once a week, because it can take a long time for too much urine to "build up" in the bladder. More often, to enable someone to be continent a catheter needs to be passed twice a day or more.

Some people are able to learn how to catheterise

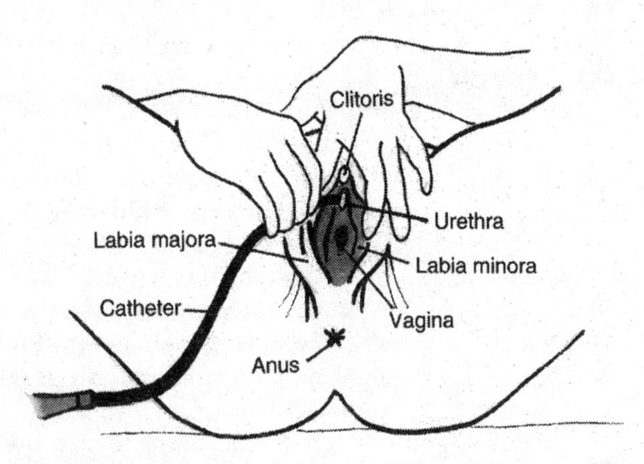

Fig 5.2 Catheter draining urine (as in intermittent catheterisation)

themselves (**self-catheterisation**), but this requires good mental ability and good use of the hands and fingers. If this is not possible then nursing staff may need to pass the catheters. In a hospital or home the catheterisation is usually performed as an "aseptic" or sterile procedure.

Intermittent catheterisation has the benefit of providing complete continence for some people and also helps to reduce urine infections because the stale urine in the bladder is removed. But it is not a suitable treatment for people with dementia or those who have other problems with brain functioning and cannot fully understand or cooperate. Sometimes the tablet used in urge incontinence (oxybutynin) is used together with intermittent catheterisation, to ensure that incontinence does not occur between catheterisations.

When overflow incontinence occurs as a result of an **obstruction** (usually an enlarged prostate gland) then an operation may be necessary to remove the obstruction. If surgery is impossible then the urine may be drained out of the bladder continuously using a permanent catheter (see chapter 6).

Providing an individualised toileting programme

For some clients, particularly people with confusion or dementia, the general toileting routine needs to be looked at. Toileting may be carried out at set times (for example before and after mealtimes, or every two hours) because it is impossible to tell when the client needs to pass urine. But this may mean that sometimes the client is taken to the toilet when she does not want to go (and therefore does not pass urine) or is taken to the toilet after being incontinent.

The aim of any individualised toileting programme is for the client to be helped to use the toilet at times when the bladder is fairly full, but before incontinence occurs. Don't start with the most incontinent client; choose someone who is not wet all the time

The usual toileting routine is continued to begin with, using the simple chart (see chapter 4)to form a **baseline**. Toilet visits that do not result in urine being passed in the toilet are marked on the chart with a cross, and the client's pad is checked every hour to see if it is wet or dry. Alternatively the special chart may be used (see chapter 4) to record this information.

After five to seven days of charting you will have a baseline (see chapter 4). Then take a good look at the chart and adjust the toileting times so that the client is taken to the toilet about half an hour before incontinence occurs, and toilet visits that do not result in urine being passed are stopped. .

Circle the new toileting times on a fresh chart. The client should then be taken to the toilet at these times (and the chart continued) for the following week. You should find that the number of times the resident is incontinent is reduced and that there are fewer unsuccessful toilet visits. Sometimes it may take several weeks to settle on the most effective programme for the client.

Individualised toileting is much more likely to reduce incontinence (if not stop it) than toileting people at set times, such as every two hours. But it must be said that some people do not seem to show any regular pattern and therefore may not benefit from this type of programme. In this case toileting at routine times may at least "catch" some of the incontinence.

Rewards and encouragement

Surprising though it may seem, incontinence can sometimes become rewarding in itself. Being incontinent can bring a lot of fuss and attention which would not otherwise happen if the client used the toilet.

This may be the case for some people with dementia

or with other problems with mental functioning (see chapter 3) and particularly those who do not otherwise receive much social contact. A plan to make incontinence less rewarding for the client may then be useful, once other possible causes of incontinence have been ruled out.

Usually such a plan will involve clearing up incontinence in a matter-of-fact way without added smiles, chat or touch so that incontinence is no longer rewarding. But taking the "attention" out of incontinence does not actually encourage continence. It is also important to have ways of **rewarding** continence.

The agreed plan could also include giving rewards and can be combined with an individualised toileting programme. The client is checked hourly or two hourly to see if the pad is dry and taken to the toilet at times indicated by their individualised programme.

If the client can indicate that she wants to use the toilet (or not) then she is reminded to go to the toilet, but only taken if she says she wishes to. If the toilet is used then the client is praised or rewarded ("That's good Mrs. Jenkins, you have used the toilet"), or if the pad is found to be dry then the client is given some special attention, perhaps a few minutes conversation and some smiles or something that the client is very keen on (maybe some food treat).

The reward should be given immediately: if there is a delay then the client may not associate the reward with the "continence". It is also important that the reward is relevant for the client – there is not much point in a food treat if the client has just had lunch and a bar of chocolate. Find out first, perhaps from relatives, what the client would regard as being rewarding. And when giving praise remember not to treat the client as a child ("Good girl, Betty"). A plan of rewards and encouragement should always be agreed (and organised) by senior staff and carried out by all staff.

Whilst it is acceptable to take the reward out of incontinence, it is not acceptable to put punishment in its place. It is very rarely possible to justify any form of punishment in residential settings.

Combining ways to improve incontinence

Other ways to improve continence will, of course, depend upon the results of the assessment. The plan of action will often involve trying to improve a number of problems. For example, a client with urge incontinence, may also have problems with hormone shortage, constipation and difficulties with slow toileting because of poor mobility and problems getting on and off the toilet.

Physiotherapy and regular walks with good footwear should improve mobility and constipation; a bladder training programme, possibly combined with oxybutynin and hormone treatment should help the bladder problem; a course of enemas, extra drinks and attention to diet will treat and prevent constipation; a pan-type urinal at night, a raised toilet seat with rails and easily removed clothing should make toileting quicker and easier. All this may add up to the client gaining continence.

KEY POINTS

- Constipation should usually be dealt with first.
- Urine infection may need to be treated.
- Urge incontinence may be helped by bladder training and/or oxybutynin.
- Stress incontinence may be improved by pelvic floor exercises and sometimes surgery.
- Overflow incontinence that is caused by nerve damage is often helped by intermittent catheterisation.
- If an obstruction is causing overflow incontinence then this may be removed by a surgical operation.
- Clients who are confused or demented may benefit from an invidualised toileting programme; this may be combined with a plan of rewards and encouragement.

6
Living with incontinence

Think positive! Products which can help: pads and pants. Bedpads. Sheaths for men. Catheters. Skin care. Hygiene. Smells. Clothes and shoes. Leading a normal life

Despite your best efforts some clients will continue to be incontinent. This may be about a quarter of clients in most homes. For some of these people you will be able to improve their incontinence, but not to get rid of it completely.

It is important not to feel that you have failed with these clients. Sometimes incontinence has to be accepted. But this does not mean that you can do no more to help. Indeed, now your job becomes even more important. You need to help your client to live with incontinence.

Being incontinent does not have to mean all the bad things we discussed in chapter 1. Many people learn to manage their problem and lead a normal life, despite being incontinent.

Think positive!

As with any other problem, "thinking positive" will make a big difference. Don't assume that any activity is impossible, just because a client is incontinent. Your attitude will often rub off on the client. If you feel that he or she cannot possibly go on a trip, go to church or stay with relatives, then the client will often think so too.

What your incontinent clients need is support and encouragement, as well as practical help and products. With careful planning and a little thought, it should be possible to hide incontinence completely.

Which products can help?

There are hundreds of different incontinence products available which are made to help keep an incontinent person comfortable and made to ensure that nobody else need know. Selecting the right product to meet individual needs is very important. Usually a trained nurse should make the assessment for this.

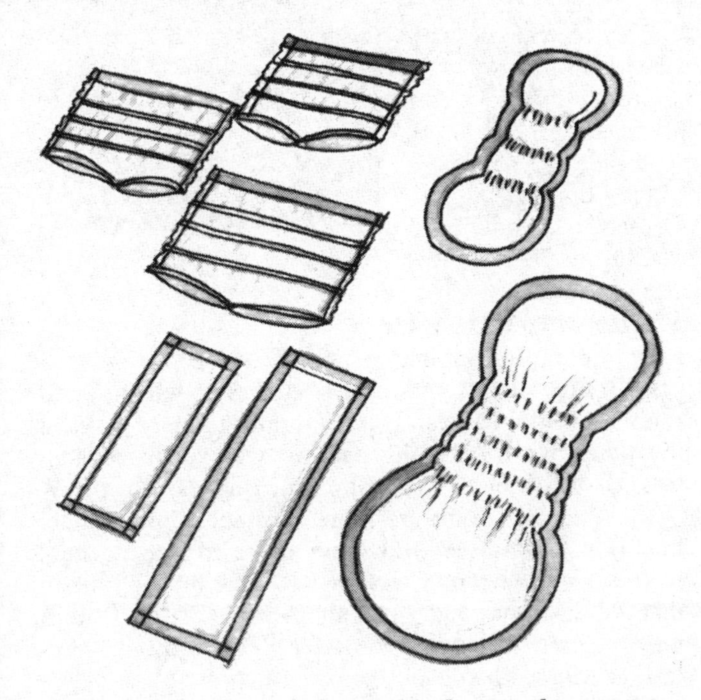

Fig 6.1 Small and large pants and pads examples.

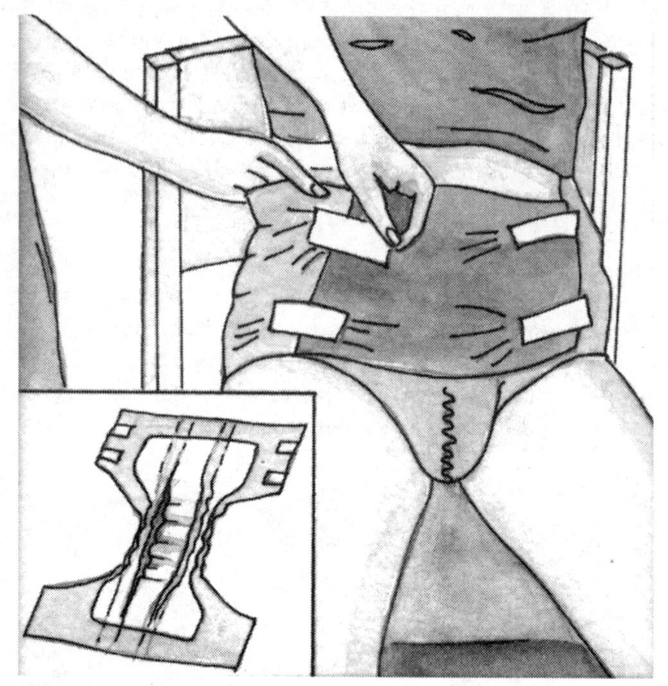

Fig 6.2 All-in-one example.

Pads and pants

People come in all shapes and sizes. So do pads and pants (Fig 6.1). The smallest one that will hide the problem is usually best. It is important to make sure that the pants worn with the pads fit well to prevent any leakage. Most pads are disposable and can be thrown away after use. Some pads are washable (only suitable for urine, not faeces) and some are sewn into washable pants. A pad and pant is easier to take off for toileting than an all-in-one pad. The all-in-ones (Fig 6.2) should only be used for very incontinent people, usually those who cannot walk at all.

It is important to put a pad on carefully. If you just

push it up between the legs, urine often runs out of the sides. If you "cup" or fold the pad first (Fig 6.3) it is less likely to leak. Some people will need a larger and more absorbent pad at night than in the day.

For men who only have a slight incontinence problem (such as dribbling urine) a penis pouch (Fig 6.4) may be preferable to pads and pants.

Bed pads

If the client wears pads and pants in bed there may be no need for a bedpad. Sometimes a thin bedpad is used as a back-up, but these often "ruck up" in the bed and are uncomfortable and ineffective. Often a simple draw sheet is better than a thin pad. Other people do not wear

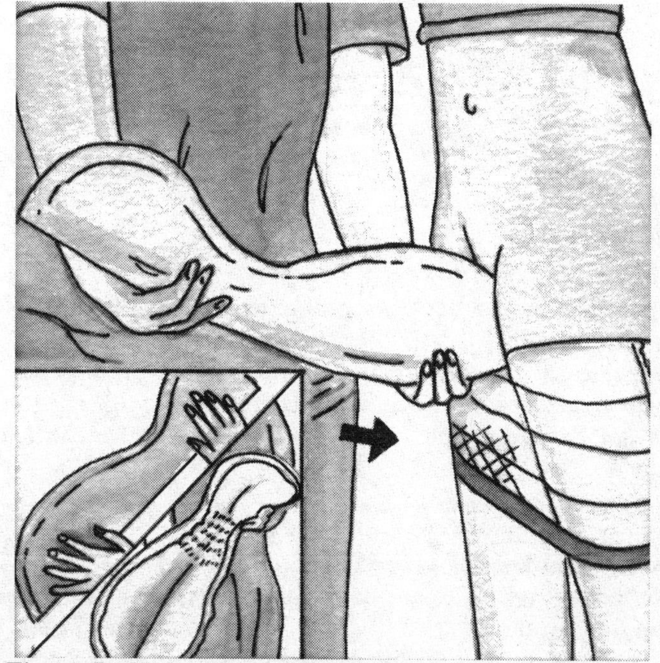

Fig 6.3 Pad being "cupped" ready for use.

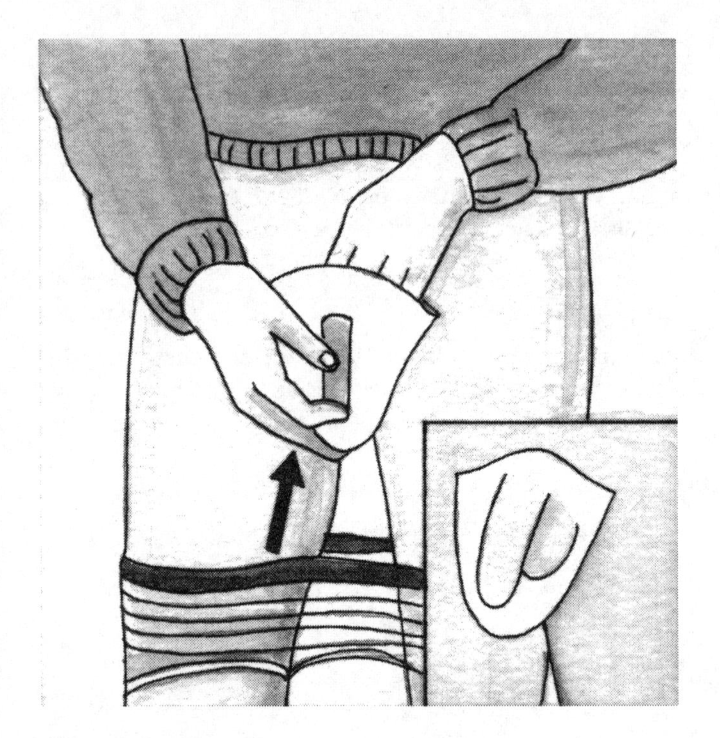

Fig 6.4 Penis pouch.

a pad, but have a thick disposable or washable bed pad. Some of the big pads (either bedpads or pads worn with pants) hold enough urine to allow the client a good night's sleep without needing a change. But you should always change people with sore skin or faecal incontinence as soon as possible.

Sheaths for men

Some men prefer to use a sheath (sometimes called a condom urinal) instead of a pad. The sheath fits closely over the penis and is connected to a leg bag which col-

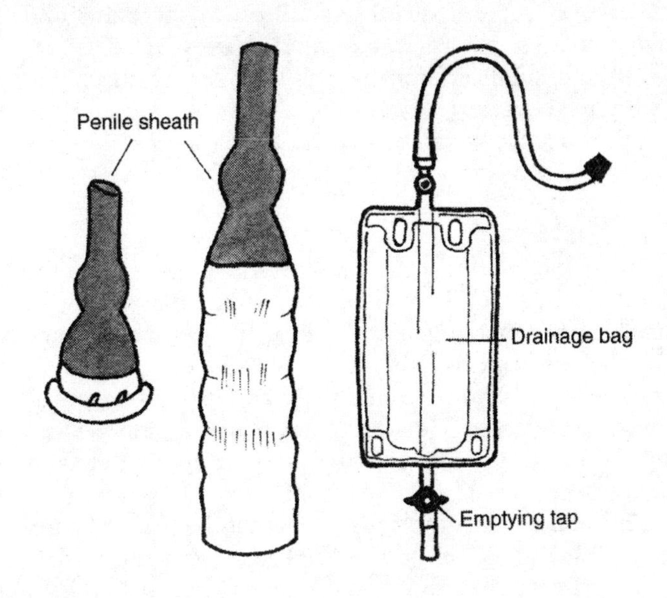

Fig 6.5 Sheath with leg bag. Tube fits into sheath tip.

lects the urine (Fig 6.5). A larger bedside bag can be used at night. Some sheaths are sticky themselves, others need to be used with a strip of adhesive on the penis.

Men who have a very small penis will not usually be able to keep a sheath on. Some confused men may pull the sheath off. But many men do prefer a sheath to a pad, and it is usually worth a try.

There are a few simple rules when using a sheath. The skin will need to be washed and thoroughly dried before the sheath is put on. It will not stick properly to wet skin, nor to creams or talcum powder, so do not use these. Long pubic hairs will need to be trimmed as they get stuck to the sheath. Use the manufacturer's measuring device to make sure that you get the right size. Follow the instructions for putting the sheath on and make sure that the sheath is well on to the penis and that it is stuck all the way around. **Never** use a sheath that is too small or tight as this can cut off the blood supply to the penis, which can be very dangerous. Each sheath is usually worn for a day and then changed.

Catheters

A catheter is a hollow tube which drains urine from the bladder into a bag. It may be fitted in the bladder outlet (urethral catheter, Fig 6.6) or in through the abdomen (supra-pubic catheter, Fig 6.7). A catheter should only be used for incontinence if all else has failed to keep the client comfortable. But for some people a catheter can allow them to go out without worrying about toilets or incontinence.

The skin around the catheter should be washed carefully each day. Soap and water is fine and there is no reason why clients cannot have a bath if they would have one normally. A leg bag should be used in the day as it can be hidden under clothes. Usually men will have a

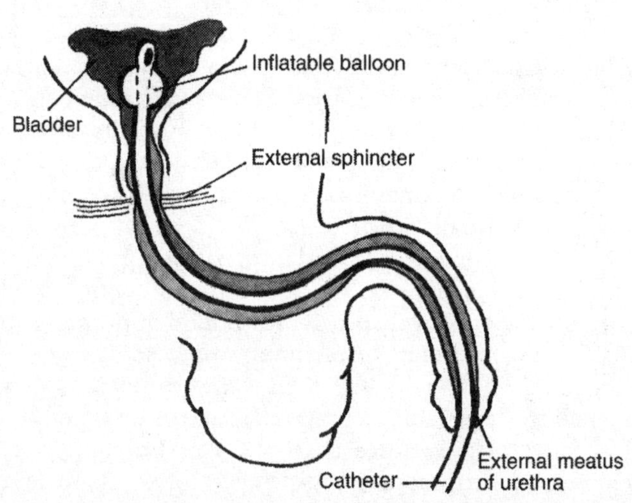

Fig 6.6 Catheter fitted in the bladder outlet (urethra).

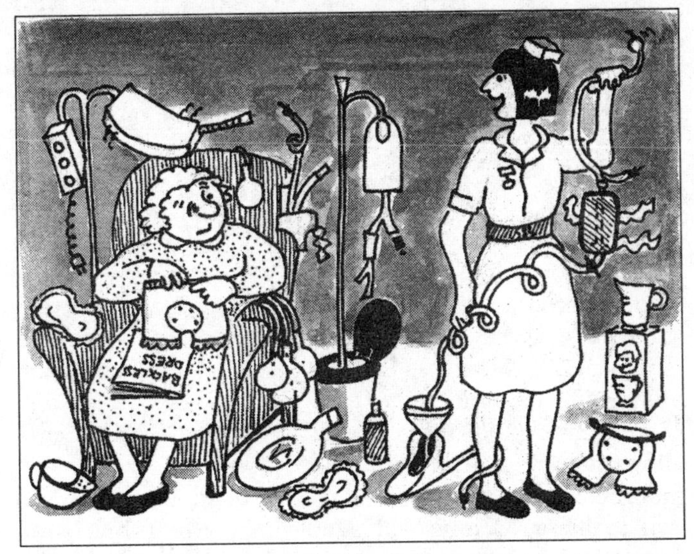

There is a wide range of aids and equipment to manage incontinence.

bag on their calf and women will have a bag on their thigh. Make sure that the leg bag straps are used according to the manufacturer's instructions so that they are comfortable and not too tight. Special garments are available as an alternative to straps.

Leg bags come with different types of taps for emptying the bag and some are easier to open than others. If possible the client should have a bag that they can empty independently. A larger bag can be connected to the tap at the end of the bag during the night.

A leg bag should last about a week and then be changed for a new one. If you change the bag always wash your hands before and after, wear gloves and do not touch the tip of the new leg bag or the very end of the catheter. Sometimes bladder washouts may be given on the advice of a nurse or doctor, to stop the catheter getting blocked.

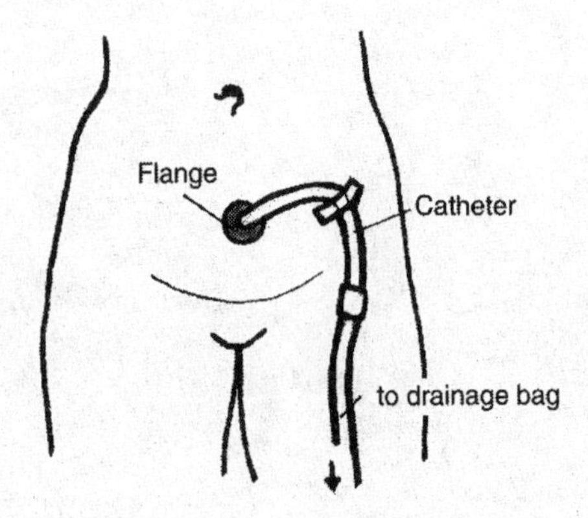

Fig 6.7 Catheter fitted in the abdominal wall.

Some clients can be shown how to look after their own catheter. Others will need your help. When you empty the bag use plastic gloves and a clean jug for each bag. Always wash your hands carefully before and after touching the catheter or bag so that you do not spread infection from one client to another. A trained nurse will usually change the catheter every two to three months.

Encourage a client with a catheter to drink plenty. At least three pints a day is best. If no urine drains from the catheter for a few hours a nurse should be told.

Skin care

Most people who are incontinent do not get sore skin, as long as the pads are changed often and the skin is washed and dried well. People who cannot move much on their own are most at risk of soreness. Sometimes a pad or sheath is rubbing. Or the person is generally not very well.

Most people do not need any cream, but if the client is sore, a simple barrier cream (like zinc and castor oil) or a cream for urine rash (such as Sudocrem) may help.

Hygiene

To help prevent any infections spreading from one client to another remember to wash your hands after you have dealt with incontinence or touched anything wet with urine. Always wash your hands after attending to clients. Check your home or hospital's policy on wearing gloves.

Wet or soiled linen needs to be placed in the correct laundry bag and wet pads must be disposed of in bags for clinical waste (check with your manager if you are not sure where wet linen or soiled rubbish should go). Seal bags as soon as possible to prevent smells.

On trips or journeys it may be useful to take sealable plastic bags (such as freezer bags) for keeping wet pads until they can be disposed of. Good hygiene will help prevent problems with smell in your hospital or home and is essential for controlling infection.

Smells

Fresh urine should not smell nasty. If it does, there may be an infection and a urine sample should be tested. Urine only starts to smell if it is left out in the air. So the best way to stop smells from incontinence is to change the client as soon as possible and to use the right continence aid so that urine does not get onto the chairs, carpet or bed. Fresh air in a room is one of the best ways of getting rid of any smell.

Smell from faecal incontinence is less easy to hide. There are some special deodorants available in chemists which can help to absorb smells.

Clothes and shoes

If the right product is used clothes and shoes should not get wet or soiled very often. But if they do, it is a good idea to choose clothes that are easy to wash and iron. Dark colours tend to show wet patches less than light colours. Shoes are usually easier to clean than slippers (unless the slippers are washable) and are often better for walking.

Leading a normal life

Careful selection of the best product for the client will ensure that she feels comfortable and confident and that nobody else knows about the problem.

With a little thought and planning even those clients who remain incontinent can be helped to lead a normal and active life.

KEY POINTS

- Continence is not possible for everyone.
- Pads and pants are available in different sizes and may be disposable or washable; all-in-ones are more difficult for toileting.
- Men often prefer a sheath with a leg-bag instead of pads and pants.
- If other aids are not successful, a catheter and leg-bag may be used.
- Good hygiene is essential to help prevent the spread of infection.
- Effective aids should stop urine from getting on to carpets and furniture and prevent smell.
- Careful selection of good quality aids will help clients to feel confident and secure and enable them to join in social activities.

7

A final word

Summary. Glossary. Sources of information and help. Further reading. Pelvic floor exercises.

Taking on the challenge of helping clients maintain and regain continence is more than just worthwhile, it is good for clients and good for you. Be positive. As we saw in chapter 2, incontinence is not inevitable for someone who lives in a residential setting such as a home. Many people can be helped to be continent, and your knowledge and skills can make the difference.

Assessing incontinence (chapter 4) is the key to finding out what is causing the problem, so that effective treatment can be given (chapter 5). If incontinence persists then good aids will ensure that clients can live their lives with confidence and dignity (chapter 6).

The care you give, based on the sound practice set out in this book, can make a huge contribution to your clients' independence and enjoyment of life.

Glossary

ANUS. The back passage where faeces come out.

BLADDER. Balloon-shaped organ which stores urine. It lies just behind the pubic bone.

COCCYX. Tail bone at the bottom of the spine.

CYSTITIS. Infection of the bladder and urine. There is often pain or burning when passing urine, and the urine may smell nasty, be cloudy or be coloured slightly red from the blood in it.

DIURETICS. "Water tablets". Often prescribed by the doctor for people with heart or breathing problems. Diuretics make you produce more urine.

FAECES. The waste product from food after it has passed through the bowel. Faeces are stored in the rectum and passed out through the anus. Most people pass a bowel motion between three times a day and three times a week. A normal bowel motion should be formed in a lump, and be soft and easy to pass without straining.
Other words your client might use: poo, bowel motions, shit, number twos, crap.

IMPACTED. If a person is very constipated the rectum can become very full and the faeces may become hard and dry.

INCONTINENCE. Inability to control the passing of urine or faeces.

PELVIC FLOOR. A hammock of muscles from beneath the pubic bone to the coccyx, which helps to keep the anus and urethra closed.

PROSTATE GLAND. Grows around the bladder outlet in men. The prostate grows larger in all men over 50 years old, and can start to block the bladder outlet.

PUBIC BONE. Bone at the bottom front of the body, behind the pubic hair.

RECTUM. Part of the bowel just above the anus, where faeces are stored.

URETHRA. Bladder outlet. The urethra opens at the end of the penis in men and just in front of the vagina in women.

URGENCY. Having to rush to pass urine or faeces.

URINE. Pale straw-coloured liquid, produced by the kidneys to get rid of some of the body's waste chemicals and water. Urine is stored in the bladder. It should not smell unpleasant (and if it does it may be infected). Most people make 2-3 pints (1,000-1,500 mls) in 24 hours, and pass urine 4-7 times a day.
Other words your client might use: pee, wee, number ones, piss, water, piddle, jimmy riddle.

VAGINA. Birth canal in women.

Sources of help and information

The Continence Foundation is a charity which provides information and education for professionals and the public. An **Incontinence Information Helpline** is staffed by continence advisors Monday-Friday 2-7pm. Tel: 0191 213 0050. A **Continence Resource Pack** has been prepared for the primary health care team (free, but please send £1 to cover P&P).

The Continence Foundation,
The Basement
2 Doughty Street
London WC1N 2PH
Tel: 0171 404 6875.

InconTact is an organisation for people with continence problems and their carers.

InconTact,
2 Doughty Street,
London WC1N 2PH.

Relatives Association. An organisation for relatives of people in homes.

The Relatives Association
5 Tavistock Place
London WC1H 9SS.
Tel: 0171 916 6055.

Several other charities provide information specific to their client group. These include:

Spinal Injuries Association
Newpoint House
76 St James's Lane, London N10 3DF.
Tel: 0181 444 2121.
Counselling line 0181 883 4296 (open 2-5pm, Monday to Friday).

Alzheimer's Disease Society,
Gordon House,
10 Greencoat Place
London SW1P 1PH.
Tel: 0171 306 0606.

ASBAH
(Association for Spina Bifida and Hydrocephalus),
Asbah House,
42 Park Road,
Peterborough PE1 2UQ.
Tel: 01733 555988.

Multiple Sclerosis Society of Great Britain and Northern Ireland,
25 Effie Road,
Fulham,
London SW6 1EE.
Tel: 0171 736 6267.

Stroke Association
CHSA House
123-127 Whitecross Street,
London EC1Y 8JJ.
Tel: 0171 490 7999.

Further reading

Understanding incontinence, by Dorothy Mandelstam (Chapman and Hall, London).

In control - help with incontinence, by Penny Mars (Age Concern, London).

Nursing for continence, by Christine Norton (Beaconsfield Publishers). Textbook for nurses and other carers.

Incontinence and inappropriate urinating, by Graham Stokes (Winslow Press, Bicester). Advice on helping confused incontinent people.

Learning to do pelvic floor exercises

Chapter 3 describes the muscles of the pelvic floor (p41). It is important for all women to learn how to do these exercises to help prevent incontinence.

1. Sit comfortably with your knees slightly apart. Now imagine that you are trying to stop yourself passing wind from the bowel. To do this you must squeeze the muscle around the back passage. Try squeezing and lifting that muscle as if you really do have wind. You should be able to feel the muscle move. Your buttocks and legs should not move at all. You should be aware of the skin around the back passage tightening and being pulled up and away from your chair. Really try to feel this.

2. Now imagine that you are sitting on the toilet passing urine. Picture yourself trying to stop the stream of urine. Really try to stop it. Try doing that now as you are reading this. You should be using the same group of muscles that you used before, but don't be surprised if you find this harder than exercise 1.

3. Next time you go to the toilet to pass urine, try the 'stop test' about half way through emptying your bladder. Once you have stopped the flow of urine, relax again and allow the bladder to empty completely. You may only be able to slow down the stream.

Don't worry; your muscles will improve and strengthen with time and exercise. If the stream of urine speeds up when you try to do this exercise, you are squeezing the wrong muscles.

Do not get into the habit of doing the "stop test" every time you pass urine. This exercise should be done only once a day at the most.

PRACTISING YOUR EXERCISES

1. Sit, stand or lie with your knees slightly apart. Slowly tighten and pull up the pelvic floor muscles as hard as you can. Hold tightened for at least 5 seconds if you can, then relax. Repeat at least five times. (Slow pull-ups).

2. Now pull the muscles up quickly and tightly, then relax immediately. Repeat at least five times. (Fast pull-ups).

3. Do these two exercises - five slow and five fast - at least 10 times every day.

4. As the muscles get stronger, you will find that you can hold for longer than 5 seconds, and that you can do more than five pull-ups each time without the muscle getting tired.

5. It takes time for exercise to make muscles stronger. You are unlikely to notice improvement for several weeks - so stick at it! You will need to exercise regularly for several months before the muscles gain their full strength.

Index